Baby Blueprints

Acupuncture and genetic testing
before
you get pregnant
plus modern options with IVF

by Karen Reynolds,
L.Ac., M.S., R.N.

ISBN: 978-1-943775-00-2

CONTENTS

Welcome to
Baby Blueprints!

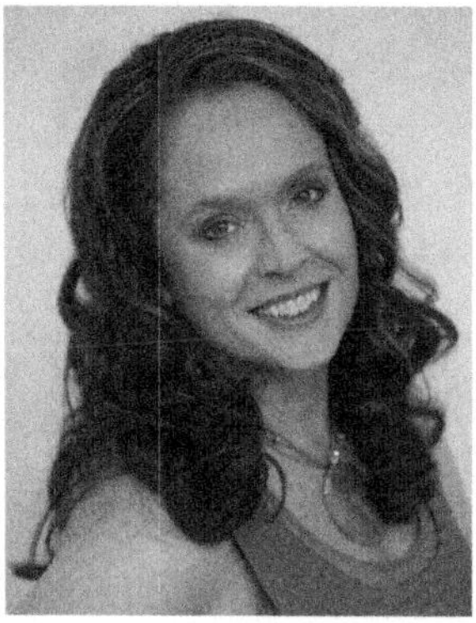

My name is Karen Reynolds. I have been a critical care RN for 26 years, and I am also a state-licensed acupuncturist, practicing in Corte Madera, California. During the past 15 years, I have specialized in fertility issues for both men and women. By combining my conventional medical experience with my experience using acupuncture and Chinese herbs, I have the honor of treating thousands of people, many of whom become pregnant and are parents to happy, healthy babies. I also work all too often with people who face genetic challenges and must therefore make some big decisions which go along with those challenges.

This book, *Baby Blueprints,* shares with you some unique and safe ways you can take specific steps towards a healthy pregnancy. *Baby Blueprints* pairs cutting-edge fertility medicine and genetic testing options with classic, 3,000 year old Chinese acupuncture procedures to produce positive results. Odd though this may be, every day I use both approaches when I treat my patients.

The decision to have a child is a big one for you, your partner, your family, and your own medical team members. Being a science nerd in my heart of hearts, I have actively researched testing options within the emerging field of human genetics. If you are considering becoming pregnant, I want to share with you what I have learned, even if you have already have children or if you simply want to test or investigate your options. There are exciting, valuable options out there for you.

If you are actively trying to get pregnant or contemplating this, I strongly recommend genetic testing for both parents ***before*** conception. Yes, some forms of genetic testing can be done only once a pregnancy is underway, such as blood and ultrasound testing 11-13 weeks into the pregnancy to rule out Down's syndrome. But affordable genetic tests, which rule out many inherited diseases, are now available ***before*** you become pregnant. This is enormously important to prospective parents, especially if there is any family history of cystic fibrosis, Tay-Sachs disease, thalassemia, or sickle cell anemia. In the later chapters I also discuss another aspect of genetic testing that takes place in the context of an assisted reproductive laboratory setting, such as in vitro fertilization. There are special cases where a single cell can be pulled from an embryo to detect cystic fibrosis or inherited genetic conditions such as breast, ovarian, and bowel cancers.

Baby Blueprints additionally includes information on what is known as "direct to consumer" (DTC) genetic testing products. There is ample discussion within the medical research and ethics community as well as the consumer world about the availability and use of these types of tests. Genetic topics are complex, personal and more complicated that you may think. Please remember there are pros, cons, bonuses, and limitations concerning all types of testing.

When making health decisions, it is wise to draw information from a clinically experienced team of medical professionals. This is one reason why I strongly recommend seeing a genetic counselor before doing any sort of testing. The chapter on genetic counseling includes an interview with genetics counselor Amy Vance. The Modern Genetics chapter includes an interview with Dr. Christo Zouves, of the Zouves Fertility Center in Foster City, California. Dr. Zouves has an on site fully accredited genetics lab and offers the most up to date genetic testing associated with in vitro fertilization treatment.

We are living in a blessed time. We have so many options and so many rich paths of information available to us. There is wisdom in exploration, consideration, and selection of the right choice for you. There is wisdom in making an educated decision, having weighed all the known possibilities. What does your heart hold dear? It will be different for each person.

After reading this book, you may decide that genetic testing is something of value to you or you may decide against it. My intention is to enable you to make the most educated choice. There is no one "right" way or "right" single course of action for all persons. I invite you to read, digest, and consider all aspects of this in your heart of hearts and use it to the best and greatest good for you, your family, and all of those you love.

CHAPTER

1

CARRIER TESTING:

Traditional, Evolving, and Why to Consider it *Before* Pregnancy

CARRIER TESTING

Traditional, Evolving, and Why to Consider it *Before* Pregnancy

Humans inherit genes in pairs from our biological parents—one from our mother and one from our father. In many instances, even if you inherit one gene with a mutation or genetic abnormality, the other healthy gene will be responsible for functioning. So it is quite common for a person to carry a gene mutation but not have any physiological issues. However, genetically inherited health problems do show up if a child happens to inherit two mutated genes, one from each parent.

Very generally speaking, if two recessive gene carrier parents have children, there is approximately a one in four (25%) chance that the child will be affected. If one dominant gene carrier parent has children, there is a 50% chance that the child will be affected.

Being a carrier (of recessively inherited diseases) means that an individual has no physical symptoms or health complaints but does carry one copy of a problematic gene, which could be passed on to children. Traditional genetic screening prior to becoming pregnant will determine if you or your mate is a carrier for common genetic disorders.

Testing can definitely give rise to anxiety, so it is important to keep in mind that just because a person has a particular gene, it does not necessarily mean that they will absolutely develop disease or pass on disease to a child. Many variables come into play within the delicate strands of DNA in our highly complex human bodies. To illustrate, the *Journal of the American Medical Association* (JAMA), a well-respected peer reviewed medical journal, says, "... the belief that genetics completely determines phenotypic outcome must be informed by an understanding that most genetic measurements only shift the probability of an outcome, which often depends on other environmental triggers and chance."[1]

This is a fancy way of saying that genes do not always translate to sure future occurrences. Many factors, not only gene makeup, determine your baby's health. Knowing that the possibility of a health problem may be present in the future for you or your child can be a valuable opportunity to prepare now and take measures to stay as healthy as possible. Results are not simply black or simply white.

There is great support for genetic testing among well-respected professional organizations. Some of these include the American Congress of Obstetricians and Gynecologists (ACOG), the American College of Medical Genetics and Genomics (ACMG) and the Ashkenazi Jewish Panel (AJ).

For 15 years, former director of the National Institutes of Health, Dr. Francis S. Collins, directed the National Human Genome Research Institute and led the Human Genome Project to its successful completion. It goes without saying that I trust his professional and clinical opinion. In his book, *The Language of Life*, Dr. Collins states, "...genes are generally not destiny, especially for common conditions like heart disease, diabetes, or cancer."[2] An amazing thing about knowing your genome and your possible risks is that in many instances, you can take specific measures to help keep those risk genes asleep rather than "switched on" in your system.

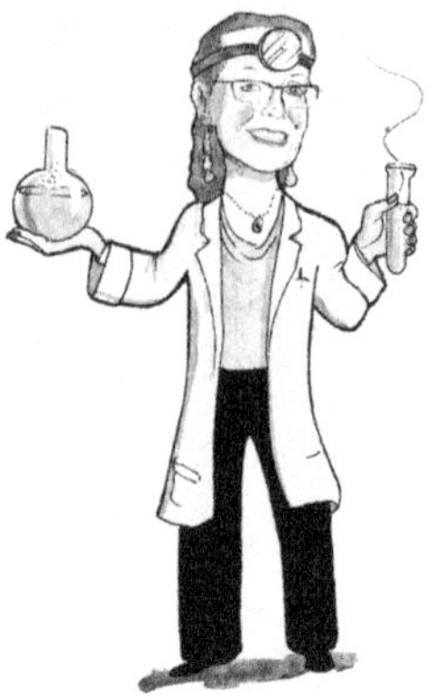

Science Nerd Corner:

"Genotype" refers to your particular genetic constitution, for example, your unique cells.

"Phenotype" refers to how your genes interact with your environment and is often intimately related to how you take care of yourself. Some genes can even remain dormant, so to speak, when measures are taken to optimize nutrition, rest, exercise and reduction of daily stressors.

"Genome" refers to your overall genetic blueprint, for example, the grand plan, which holds your complete set of genes.

Genetic Testing Before Becoming Pregnant?

If you are actively trying to get pregnant or considering it, I strongly recommend meeting with a genetic counselor to discuss the recommended genetic testing for both parents *before* becoming pregnant. Standard genetic screening is often not proposed until a pregnancy is well under way, but knowledge about this before pregnancy can be pivotal in your family planning.

Completing a thorough and professional family history is key to finding this information. This is another process best undertaken with a genetic counselor. You will find more on this topic later in the book.

To Test or Not to Test

There are, of course, reasonable and weighty concerns about the right to decline genetic testing when you are pregnant. I respect these personal decisions always. If you are inclined to forego genetic testing prior or during pregnancy because you will never terminate a pregnancy under any conditions, please consider the following. Prior knowledge of the possibility of having a special needs child can help you prepare for this occurrence.

This discussion reminds me of a dear friend of mine. She and her husband are deeply religious and opted not to have any genetic testing before the birth of their son. They also knew they would never contemplate terminating a pregnancy. Their child was born with severe spina bifida. They have no regrets. Their child is happy and his parents regard him as a great gift. However, the stress they experienced amid the shock learning of his disease, paired with the immense requirements for his health care immediately after birth, were enormous. If this book can lessen the burden of pain I saw my friends endure, then this book has accomplished my primary intention.

I have seen great anguish, shock, and heartache after births in which simple carrier testing would have afforded the prospective parents an easier transition. Special needs children usually require modified home settings and training in their physical care. For example, it can be invaluable to meet and speak with parents of special needs children and to learn how to develop a support system for yourself and your family. With this preparation and support, you can then welcome your new baby into a community and family with open arms and a good foundation of knowledge.

Standard Carrier Testing on the Beaten Path: Cystic Fibrosis, Tay-Sachs Disease, Thalassemia, and Sickle-cell disease

Hereditary Diseases in Common Populations

Cystic fibrosis	Northern European
Tay-Sachs disease	Ashkenazi Jewish
Thalassemia	Mediterranean or Southeast Asian
Sickle-cell anemia	West African

Cystic Fibrosis

In contrast to Down syndrome, we know that cystic fibrosis (CF) is a genetically inherited disease usually discovered in infancy. With CF there is a malfunction or a "misspelling" of a particular gene. The CF gene malfunction leads to cysts or scarring of the pancreas and, in turn, a lack of digestive enzymes the pancreas produces. Very thick, sticky phlegm in the lungs also develops and predisposes the child to many lung infections. The phlegm also can block the pancreas, and it typically causes nutritional problems with absorption. Blocked intestines early in infancy can point toward a CF diagnosis.

People sometimes take comfort in a quick glance at their immediate and extended family, not noting any family members with health issues. In the case of recessive genes, such as the ones that cause cystic fibrosis, those genes may be passed along for many generations with no one showing any signs of illness. You can be a carrier and not have any signs or symptoms of disease. Your siblings and parents can also be carriers and still be healthy. There are differences in how recessive genes and dominant genes are passed. If you want to further explore the differences between recessive genetic diseases and dominant genetic diseases you can easily find this information on the Internet.

As a pregnant woman, you will likely not be tested for being a carrier of CF until your first prenatal visit with your doctor; however, by that time your pregnancy is well under way. It is easy, inexpensive, and wise to have carrier testing for CF done *before* falling pregnant. The following table lists the probabilities for cystic fibrosis in a child born to parents for whom both are CF gene carriers.

Cystic Fibrosis Risk If Both Parents Are Carriers

3-in-4 chance (75%) that a baby born to these two parents will not have CF

1-in-2 chance (50%) that at baby born to these two parents will NOT have CF but, like the parents, will be a carrier for the CF gene

1-in-4 (25%) chance that a baby born to these two parents will have CF

1-in-4 (25%) chance that a baby born to these two parents will NOT have CF and will NOT be a carrier for the CF gene

Tay-Sachs Disease

The screening for Tay-Sachs disease—also a genetically inherited condition—is handled and timed quite differently. Tay-Sachs disease is found primarily in individuals of East European Jewish (Ashkenazi) background. Infants born with Tay-Sachs are missing an enzyme called hexosaminidase. At birth, the children appear normal. However, as waste products build in the baby's system, blindness, deafness, and paralysis ensue. Children with Tay-Sachs generally do not survive beyond 4 or 5 years of age. In the 1970s there was great interest within the Jewish communities for screening, and an enzyme test was created. The Jewish communities have readily embraced and instituted pre-pregnancy screening, which affords couples other planning options.

Thalassemia

Thalassemia is an inherited disorder in which a baby has a greatly reduced ability to make hemoglobin. Hemoglobin is the protein component of red blood cells, which carries oxygen to body tissues and carbon dioxide away from body tissues. All cells in our bodies require adequate amounts of oxygen every minute of every day. Without enough hemoglobin, the body will suffer from anemia and make very small red blood cells, which cannot carry the usual amount of oxygen. Normal hemoglobin levels in the body range somewhere from 12.5g/dL to 16g/dL. A person with thalassemia may have hemoglobin ranging from 10.5g/dL to as low as 6g/dL.

Because they cannot make hemoglobin, children with thalassemia require regular blood transfusions to provide the needed oxygen for their bodies. Without transfusions, they will develop bone damage, bone pain, growth abnormalities, enlarged spleen, and higher pressures within their lungs (aka pulmonary hypertension), and heart failure. Iron overload becomes a problem for these children as well because each bag of transfused blood typically contains 200-250mg of iron, and the body has no natural way to get rid of large amounts of iron.

Chelators are a must for anyone with thalassemia. These are drugs, which help remove iron or block iron absorption in the body. According to Dr. Thomas D. Coates of Children's Hospital in Los Angeles, if chelators are taken daily and consistently, it is an effective way to remove iron from the body. There will be fewer complications of thalassemia, and a near normal life expectancy is projected. However, compliance with intake of the chelators proves to be an enormous challenge.[3]

Children with thalassemia will always require frequent blood and tissue testing as well as regularly timed medical monitoring such as specialty MRI scans to check iron concentrations.

Sickle-Cell Disease

Sickle-cell Disease is yet another inherited condition in which the red blood cells are misshapen. Usually red blood cells look rather like a doughnut with a small depression in the center. They have smooth, round edges, which easily tumble through blood vessels. In sickle-cell disease, the red blood cells are more crescent moon or sickle shaped, giving them pointy edges. Sickled red blood cells do flow around curves well. They easily clog vessels, stack up, and distort blood flow to organs and all areas of the body. This causes repeated bouts of fevers, swellings, infections and extreme pain.

Healthy red blood cells will live about 120 days, whereas sickled red blood cells only have a 10-20 day lifetime. What this means is that the bone marrow is perpetually struggling to make more red blood cells and the cells it manufactures are not healthy ones. This is why people with sickle-cell disease most always have high levels of fatigue, pain as well as what is called sickle cell anemia. At this time, sickle-cell disease is managed with medication and blood transfusions.

The National Institutes of Health state that sickle-cell disease affects between 70,000-80,000 Americans. It is estimated that it occurs in 1 in 500 African Americans and 1 in 1,000-1,400 Hispanic Americans.[4]

It is a common misconception that sickle-cell disease occurs only within African American populations. However, if you have ancestry from Mediterranean areas such as Greece, Turkey, Italy, the Arabian Peninsula, India, South America, Central America or parts of the Caribbean, you may also be at risk for being a carrier. If you have inherited one sickle-cell gene from a parent and the other inherited gene is healthy, you will not have any symptoms of the disease. However, this does mean you have what is called "sickle-cell trait" and are a carrier. This means you can pass the gene to your children.

Carrier Testing–Edging Toward the Path: The Case for Adding Spinal Muscular Atrophy and Fragile X Syndrome to Screening Panels

Spinal Muscular Atrophy

Spinal muscular atrophy (SMA) is a disease that many doctors are lobbying to be added to genetic screening panels. Infants with SMA develop loss of muscle tone over the first few months of life. This ultimately progresses to complete paralysis and death usually by age two. Approximately one in 40 people are SMA carriers but are not symptomatic themselves. This translates to a statistic of one in 1,600 pregnancies that result in a child born with SMA.[5] Another way to interpret this is there will be a one in four chance (or 25%) that children born to two carrier parents will have SMA. This is the case even if two parents have other children who do not have the disease.[6]

Unlike testing for Down syndrome, SMA testing only needs to be completed once. Genetic testing for this disease is somewhat complicated, which makes testing more costly. (At the time of this writing, a general cost estimate for SMA testing is $350-$500.) Some insurance policies will cover a portion of the testing, so out of pocket cost may be as low as $99.

A Reuters article published in 2010 discusses two sides of debate about SMA testing being added to routine prenatal screening. One side states that 12,500 women would have to be tested for SMA to detect one child with the disease, i.e., one in 10,000 pregnancies are impacted. From a health economics perspective, the authors suggest that a $500 test would not be cost effective to carry out on all 12,500 women.[7]

The American College of Genetics takes a different view, stating that the analytic tool used in the research study to calculate cost/benefit was not the ideal tool. Their study used the statistical calculation used for cystic fibrosis. Persons with CF live comparatively longer than a child with SMA, so they incur greater medical costs over time. Costs for SMA testing would easily rival medical costs over the lifetime of a child with CF. The American College of Genetics stated that the forecast of medical care costs compared with the test costs was not an accurate comparison.

Dr. Francis Collins cites in his book (also published in 2010) that one in 1,600 pregnancies results in a SMA diagnosis, thus there are some rather large statistical discrepancies to consider.[8] A one in 1,600 risk is radically higher than one in 10,000.

So, yes, a debate exists about SMA testing being routinely added to carrier screenings. I recommend discussion with a genetics counselor about adding this test to your screening panel.

Fragile X Syndrome

Fragile X syndrome is another carrier disease being considered for inclusion in routine screenings. Fragile X is responsible for mental retardation and is second only to Down syndrome in frequency, affecting approximately 1 in 4,000 boys. Usually males with fragile X who reach adulthood cannot live independently. It is estimated that 1/3 of the carrier females will have learning disabilities.

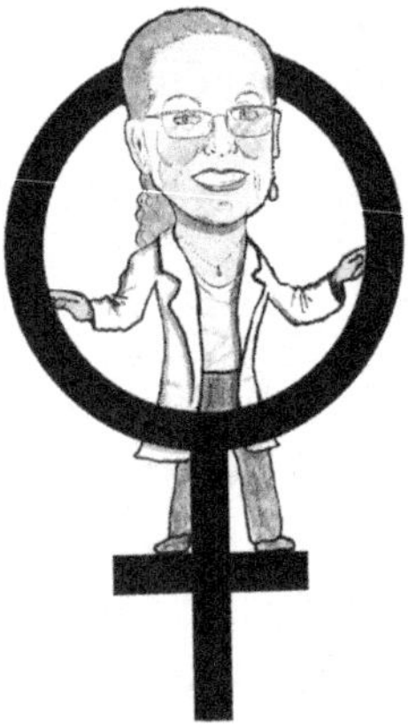

Fragile X is what is called an X-linked disease in that it can be passed on to babies when only the mother is the sole carrier of the gene mutation. Women who are carriers for fragile X have one X chromosome which is not functioning. Because females have two X chromosomes, overall they are less impacted because their healthy X chromosome will function normally. However, a woman carrying the fragile X chromosome can pass it to both male and female offspring.

One in every 259 women is a carrier for fragile X.[9] Some carrier girls are not affected; however, about 1/3 of carrier girls will have mild to moderate learning disabilities or significant intellectual challenges. Given that there is a significantly large number of carriers and given that the impacts of Fragile X can be devastating, I advise carrier screening for fragile X *before* you become pregnant.

CHAPTER

2

TYPICAL (NON-GENETIC) TESTS DURING PREGNANCY

TYPICAL (NON-GENETIC) TESTS DURING PREGNANCY

In a typical course of care at 11-13 weeks of pregnancy, a woman will be given blood tests together with an ultrasound. The blood tests measure what are called pregnancy associated plasma protein A (PAPP-A) and human chorionic gonadotropin (HCG). The ultrasound specifically seeks to check for thickness at the back of the baby's neck. Increased thickness is associated chromosome disorders. Increased HCG levels, decreased PAPP-A levels, and increased neck measurements are associated with Down syndrome.[10]

Screening for Down syndrome cannot be done until conception has occurred because 96% of Down syndrome cases are NOT considered genetically inherited situations. More specifically, with this condition there is a developmental error within the specific egg, sperm, or growing embryo. It is considered to be a random building block glitch rather than a change in the genetic code, which is passed within all cells.[11]

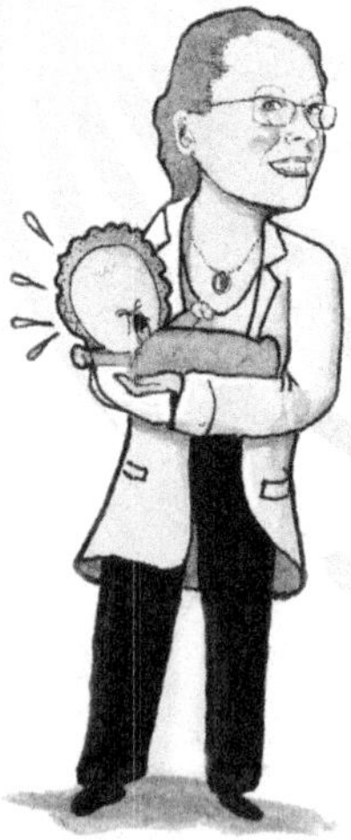

The following list, divided into five groupings, is taken from the March of Dimes Newborn Screening website. I am *not* advocating testing for all of these diseases, but I provide the list in case any of the diseases noted appear familiar to you based upon your family history.[12]

Inheritable diseases which can be genetically ruled out before becoming pregnant

1. Organic Acid Metabolism Disorders (babies with digestion problems)
   - Isovaleric acidemia (IVA)
   - Glutaric acidemia (GAI)
   - Hydroxymethylglutaric aciduria, also called 3-OH 3-CH3 glutaric aciduria (HMG)
   - Multiple carboxylase deficiency (MCD)
   - Methylmalonic acidemia, mutase deficiency (MUT)
   - 3-methylcrotonyl-CoA carboxylase deficiency (3MCC)
   - Methylmalonic academia, CB1 A and CBl B forms (Cbl A,B)
   - Propionic acidemia (PROP)
   - Beta-ketothiolase deficiency (BKT)

2. Fatty Acid Oxidation Disorders (the inability to digest fats into energy)
   - Medium-chain acyl-CoA dehydrogenase deficiency (MCAD)
   - Very long-chain acyl-CoA dehydrogenase deficiency (VLCAD)
   - Long-chain hydroxyacyl-CoA dehydrogenase deficiency (LCHAD)
   - Trifunctional protein deficiency (TFP)
   - Carnitine uptake defect (CUD)

3. Amino Acid Metabolism Disorders (Amino acids are found in proteins. There are some genetic diseases in

which a child's body either cannot break down specific amino acids for the body to use or cannot eliminate the waste products of amino acids.)

- *Phenylketonuria (PKU)*
- Maple syrup urine disease (MSUD)
- Homocystinuria (HCY)
- Citrullinemia (CIT)
- Argininosuccinic acidemia (ASA)
- Tyrosinemia type I (TYR I)

4. Hemoglobin Disorders (These problems affect red blood cells and oxygen carrying capacity in the body.)

- *Sickle cell anemia*
- *Hb S/beta-thalassemia (Hb S/Th)*
- Hb S/C disease (Hb S/C)

5. Other Disorders

- Congenital hypothyroidism (HYPOTH)
- Biotinidase deficiency (BIO)
- Congenital adrenal hyperplasia (CAH)
- Galactosemia (GALT)
- *Hearing loss (HEAR)*
- *Cystic fibrosis (CF)*
- Severe combined immunodeficiency (SCID)
- *Critical congenital heart disease (CCHD)*

How are Babies Traditionally Tested?

Currently all states require newborn genetic testing for a minimum of 26 known hereditary conditions. Forty-two states as well as the District of Columbia test for 29 genetic diseases, and the March of Dimes organization currently recommends a total of 31 tests that should be given to babies soon after birth.

Newborn Screening Tests

- Heel prick blood test to check for genetic issues
- Hearing check to make sure your baby responds to sound. Approximately 2-3 per every 1,000 babies will have a hearing impairment at birth. Speech and language development begins very early in your child's life, so if hearing is compromised it can be critical.
- An oxygen sensor applied to the finger or foot to test for how much oxygen is circulating in the blood. Lower levels can be the first indication of critical congenital heart disease (CCHD)

The heel prick test obtains several drops of blood from your baby and then tests it. The timing of getting this heel prick test differs depending upon birthing facility, hospital, etc. Usually these tests are completed within 1-2 hours after a baby is born or before leaving the hospital. For babies born outside of facilities, it is recommended they be tested within seven days of birth.

Please remember that to screen a newborn it is not enough to count ten fingers and ten toes and check for adequate breathing. Most hereditary diseases will manifest over the first few weeks or months of an infant's life even though the child initially appears normal. Today about one of every 1,000 births will result in a baby developing a disease that could have been predicted by carrier screening.

The current practice of delaying testing until pregnant can cause stressors, which might be avoided if individuals know genetic specifics before falling pregnant. Not testing before becoming pregnant also bypasses a couple's opportunity to choose preconception alternatives. Many people will want to have this information as they contemplate starting their families, so valuable conversations can take place with your doctor as well as a genetics counselor.

CHAPTER

3

TYPES OF GENETIC TESTING~HOW THEY DIFFER

TYPES OF GENETIC TESTING~HOW THEY DIFFER

Genetic tests fall into two broad types of testing: chromosome karyotyping and chromosomal microarray analysis. Microarray analysis tests are further broken down into what is called comparative genomic hybridization (CGH) or single-nucleotide polymorphism (SNP) testing. In the Modern Genetics chapter of this book, please see the interview with Dr. Christo Zouves, a reproductive endocrinologist in Foster City, California. Dr. Zouves has an on-site laboratory, which now does the newest type of genetic testing which is called "next generation sequencing."

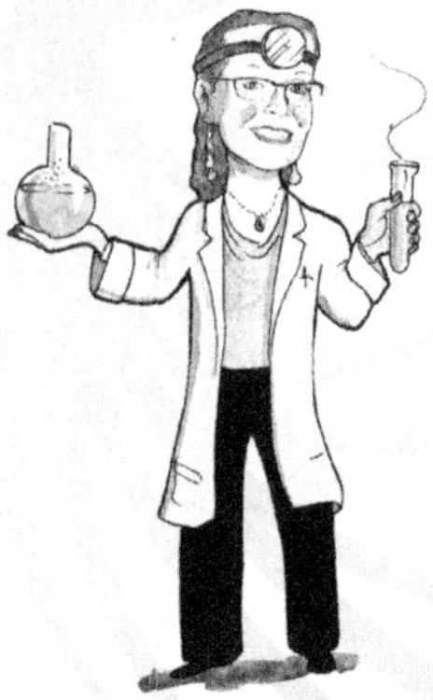

Chromosome karyotyping is often referred to in medical literature as "conventional karyotyping" because it is the older version of genetic testing. The historical beginnings of karyotyping started in the late 1800s, but the process was not fully accurate and functional until the 1950s. Karyotyping uses actively dividing cells from body from sources such as amniotic fluid, blood, bone marrow, or placenta. The cells are stained and chromosomes are photographed under high-powered microscopes. Genetic specialists then photograph the chromosomes and count them, pair them, inspect for irregularities in shape size, etc. as well as look for extra or missing chromosomes.

Limitations of Karyotype Testing

- Inability to see gene abnormalities smaller than a microscope (submicroscopic) can detect
- Requires actively dividing cells, which can limit testing in cases of investigating stillbirth or fetal demise
- Can involve human error and/or subjectivity given that it is manual counting of delicate cellular components

Compared with karyotyping, comparative genomic hybridization (CGH) is able to produce higher resolution results and thus more genetic information. It is also a standardized computerized process, so the operator error aspect is monumentally reduced. Microarray analysis is quicker because it does not require live dividing cells.

The chart below shows some examples of what are called "disclosure considerations" for chromosomal microarray testing. It is important to understand these considerations fully if you decide to pursue testing. Some of the discovery possibilities might be ones you have never imagined, and your health care team will be invaluable in helping you consider all aspects of the testing process and results.

Disclosures to Understand about Chromosomal Microarray Testing

- May discover genetic indicators of adult onset disorders, such as breast cancer, risk mutations or inherited neurological disease risk genes. The parents themselves may not show any symptoms of disease. It may be unknown how severe future disorders may be for parent and/or child.

- Will not identify all genetic disorders possible
- Will identify most genetic disorders which karyotyping would find
- May identify diseases with have a range of presentation severity. For example, disease symptoms may be minor or may be severe, and it may not be possible to predict severity
- May identify incest or non-paternity
- May identify genetic changes of uncertain significance, i.e., currently unknown if there are disease impacts or not

Prenatal parameters for chromosomal microarray testing as per the Society for Maternal-Fetal Medicine[13]

Chromosomal Microarray Analysis recommended for:

- Interested women, irrespective of maternal age, because most genetic changes found by microarray testing are not associated with older maternal age
- Ultrasound showing one or more structural abnormalities of fetus + parent(s) choosing invasive prenatal diagnosis
- Cases of still birth or intrauterine fetal demise (>20 weeks pregnancy) as a tool to detect cause

Chromosomal Microarray Analysis NOT recommended for:

- Investigation of miscarriage occurring at <20 weeks pregnancy, due to limited data on clinical utility

Chromosomal Microarray Analysis recommendations should always include:

- Documented informed consent by the patient
- Pre and post genetic counseling from a qualified genetic counselor or geneticist

In pregnancies in which ultrasounds reflect normal fetal structures, patients may choose either karyotyping OR chromosomal microarray testing.

CMA testing will discover genetic disorders such as

- Down syndrome (aka Trisomy 21)
- Patau syndrome (aka Trisomy 13)
- Edwards syndrome (aka Trisomy 18)
- Sex chromosome abnormalities
- More genetic disorders than detectable with karyotype analysis

A specimen is required when testing for chromosomal microarray. It may be taken from blood (4 ml for children or 10 ml for adults), placenta, the umbilical cord, products of conception (for example, following miscarriage), a skin biopsy, amniotic fluid (if pregnant), or a chorionic villus sample (if pregnant). Specimen processing can take 5-10 days or slightly longer and may require samples from both parents.

Depending upon the genetic disorder, reliable CMA detection rates are between 70-99%.

It is wise to remember that no test can find everything. Also keep in mind that there are some chromosomal changes that even a CMA may not find. Specialists will often recommend that couples seek both CMA testing and karyotype testing together so as to be as comprehensive as possible.

CHAPTER

4

DIRECT-TO-CONSUMER GENETIC TESTING

DIRECT-TO-CONSUMER GENETIC TESTING

In the last 10 years, accuracy and accessibility of genetic testing have exploded. You can now have genetic testing done for as little as $99 based upon a saliva test you take in the comfort and convenience of your own home. Why is this important to you as someone embarking upon getting pregnant?

The National Organization of Rare Diseases website states that there are more than 7,000 known rare diseases, which affect more than 200,000 people in the United States.[14] That might not sound like a large number of people when you consider our entire U.S. population, but rare diseases do not simply touch the person with the disease. They poignantly impact family, friends and communities. This means the number of people affected is estimated to be more than 25 million people. Knowing your genome as well as that of your mate can give you and your families invaluable planning and decision-making information.

We are living in a blessed, rich, and admittedly complex time in medical history. The technology available to us is mind-boggling compared to the options available to even our parents' generation. There are all manner of genetic tests available on the internet, but what are the reliabilities and limitations of the tests? No test is 100% infallible. Are tests checking for most commonly seen variants or mutations that pertain to you individually? How to choose? These are some questions to consider. One of my goals is to give you, the reader, a foundation from which to seek the most prudent and valuable choices for you and your family.

With respect to direct to consumer (DTC) genomic testing, the most conservative medical opinion is that this testing should be confined to use within research labs and requires more testing for validity, reliability etc. There is concern about its premature incorporation into the conventional medical setting. A more liberal medical opinion acknowledges its benefit. This is specifically noted with respect to the development of databases to make clinically relevant information useful, accessible, and applicable for medical care. There are well-respected medical groups that support easy and independent access to genetic testing and the test results. There are also equally prestigious associations that oppose access without medical supervision, etc.

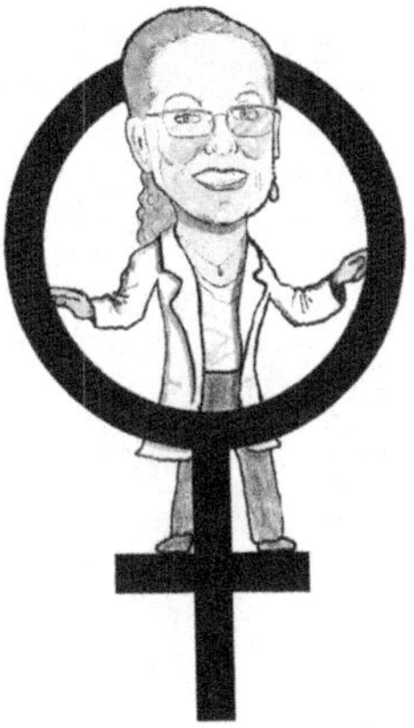

There are valid concerns within the medical community about direct-to-consumer genetic products. However, in light of genetic databases, the Committee Opinion paper number 581 from December of 2013 of The American College of Obstetricians and Gynecologists Committee on Genetics Society for Maternal-Fetal Medicine states: "...interpretation of results is expected to improve as knowledge of the human genome grows and the use of databases to link clinical findings with copy number variants becomes more robust."[15]

Genetic testing has enormous potential for drug development, treatment development, and the avoidance of unwanted or dangerous side effects of medications. My opinion is that DTC testing has value and is a tool best used in conjunction with you in consultation with both an MD and a genetic counselor. Avail yourself to the expertise of professionals who operate in these specialties and then make solid, educated decisions that are right for you.

Why my patients typically seek genetic testing before pregnancy

- Diligence around family building and planning
- Information to make informed decisions
- Concern for future generations
- Known inherited genetic issues within the family

Reasonable concerns about direct-to-consumer genetic tests

- Causing unnecessary stress or anxiety
- Not having results properly interpreted
- Seeking unnecessary medical care based upon tests
- Avoiding medical intervention when it is needed.

As I've mentioned above, debate exists within the medical community about the support of direct-to-consumer genetic testing. When searching the Internet, you'll quickly discover many websites and private companies offering testing and panels. The availability is exciting, convenient and interesting. However, there are things to consider if you opt for a direct to you product or service.

Here are additional specific pros and cons about getting testing on your own as opposed to doing so while working with an MD and/or a genetics counselor. I also give reviews of some companies and resources you may want to consider.

Ethics

Medical doctors who thoughtfully consider the ethical issues connected to the topic of genetic testing have concerns about a DNA sample being a "coded probabilistic medical record." This relates to the potentials for job or insurance discrimination based upon genetic results. DNA testing is more than just a piece of information in your medical record; it also can complicate privacy issues. The motivations to pursue tests and information independent of medical supervision are big ones, perhaps born out of curiosity, frugality, privacy or other drives. In some instances it may be fine. However, it is common for non-medical persons to consent to a test but not in fact understand the full reach of benefits, limitations, and results of that test.

Reliability

How applicable are genetic test results to your life? Areas of uncertainty exist with genetic testing. For example, it is wise to consider the reliability of various types of testing. With some gene abnormalities there are measures you can take to reduce the gene "turning on" or becoming active, so to speak. There are two genetic terms that are important to know and consider with your genetics counselor. One term is "gene penetrance" and the other one is "gene expressivity." How genes express themselves can be radically different from person to person. For example, two people with the same problematic gene may not have the same health issues or complaints.

Science Nerd Corner:

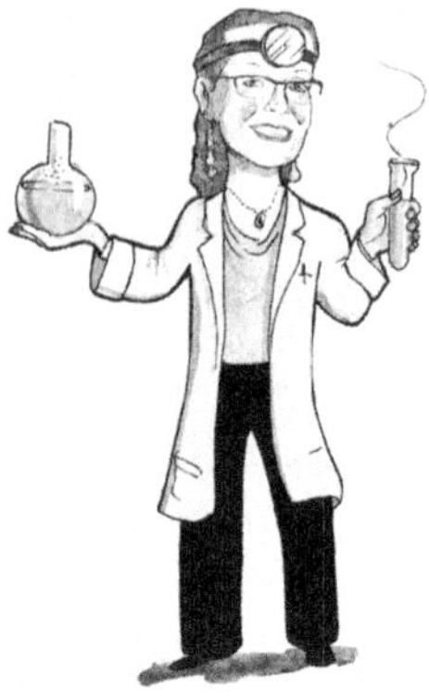

Gene penetrance refers to the portion of the population that has a disease-causing gene *and* that shows symptoms of the disease. It is comforting to know that not everyone carrying a particular gene will develop a particular disease. If, for example, a gene is associated with a 60% penetrance, this means that 60% of people carrying that gene will have disease symptoms while 40% of people carrying that same gene will not have symptoms. Knowing gene penetrance can give you a better understanding of the probability that you might develop a future issue. The penetrance varies widely for many types of diseases.

Gene expressivity essentially refers to the extent the symptoms typically are for a person carrying a disease-causing gene. For example, there might be two patients carrying the same gene mutation. Both individuals might have complaints, but one person has more complaints of greater severity than the other person.

Consents with Genetic Testing: Why is it Important to You?

All reputable laboratories, MDs, and practitioners of adjunct health care specialties will at some point require you to sign consent forms. But what do those consents really mean for you? They are not just random pieces of paper with a bureaucratic checkbox that needs to be ticked. In fact, they are a protection for you—one that you need to fully understand. When your MD orders tests, as the patient, it is your right to feel confident that the correct tests are being selected and that the results are being correctly interpreted. A full health history should be taken for you and your partner along with a review of their family histories. Practitioners should know the limits of testing and inform you of them. You also have a right to know what options are available to you in the event that a test reflects a result that requires medical care.

One point of debate raised within the medical community and the availability of DTC genetic testing concerns what is sometimes referred to as "neutral counseling." For example, there can be a conflict of interest if the party who is counseling you about genetic testing stands to gain something from you, i.e., when you purchase a test panel from them. Another popular complaint concerns risks with consumers having direct access to testing, thus bypassing medical supervision within the marketplace.[16] For example, what if a test result radically stresses out a person and the result actually is far less weighty that it might initially appear?

In contrast, what if a person truly requires medical care but does not grasp the severity of their health condition? There is concern about retail laboratories not having adequate counseling information or the ability to give proper clinical and emotional support to a consumer if a test reflects troubling results. These are concerns that medically trained practitioners worry about because ultimately MDs, counselors, acupuncturists, etc. want only safety and health for you. Another side of this argument is that some consumers need access to testing outside of their insurance policy coverage options to protect their privacy and because of fear of future discrimination.[17]

My clinical opinion is that it is wise, irrespective of who orders and runs the lab tests for you, to have proper, clinically expert support systems in place. If you choose to have genetic testing done on your own, it certainly is easily available and accessible, though it may not account for review of test reliability, pertinent family history, or future needs. Some of my clients have hired their own genetics counselor and had the tests done through private labs. Other clients have enlisted the support of their medical doctor who has ordered and interpreted tests as well as directed them to the medically recommended options.

It is always wise for your medical doctor to have a complete picture of your health when they treat you. These choices are highly personal, private, and based upon a wide range of factors. Most important is what most thoroughly serves you and your family and meets all of your needs.

Want to Find More Detailed Information about Labs and Genetic Topics?

In this section you will find links related to genetic information to further your foundation of knowledge.

http://www.ncbi.nlm.nih.gov/gtr.

At this National Institutes of Health site, you will find a genetic testing registry (GTR) of laboratories that voluntarily submit test information on the services they provide. The registry has descriptions of each test's purpose, methodology, validity, and usefulness as well as lab contact information and credentialing of those labs.

http://www.genome.gov/Glossary/

Exlpore this link for specific health conditions and more detailed clinical resources, which include the NHGRI Talking Glossary of Genetic Terms.

http://www.ncbi.nlm.nih.gov/books/NBK1116/

Gene Reviews is an online collection of chapters that describe genetic conditions (631 of them at the writing of this book). Each chapter is peer reviewed by experts in clinical genetics and laboratory genetics.

http://www.ncbi.nlm.nih.gov/medgen/

MedGen is a powerful NIH search engine specializing in human medical genetics

http://www.omim.org/

OMIM, aka Online Mendelian Inheritance in Man, provided by the Johns Hopkins University, describes itself as an online catalog of human genes and genetic disorders

http://www.orpha.net/consor/cgi-bin/index.php

Orhanet is a European consortium that serves as a portal for researching rare disease and orphan drugs

http://www.decode.com

deCode Genetics is a company located in Reykjavik, Iceland. Although deCode is no longer offering consumer genetic testing, they have an expansive website with regularly updated postings on scientific genetic findings and publications. If you are interested more technical and specific information about genetic research relevant to a particular disease, this is terrific website.

What Happens to Your DNA Specimens after Testing is Completed?

There are two camps of medical opinions regarding DNA-related samples. Some experts believe it is best for genetic samples to be immediately destroyed following testing. Others argue that there is scientific benefit in having sample collections available to benefit altruistic genetic research. This is yet another personal decision and, to that end, I always advise my clients to follow their personal preference.

Consider these questions before you decide to give a blood sample:

- How will the samples be used in the lab?
- Will the samples be used only for the test I am ordering?
- Will they be destroyed at some point when testing is completed and if so, when?
- Will any samples be used for further research, development or testing? If this answer is "yes," information should be available to you pertaining to the purposes, limits, and outcomes of that testing. There should also be information about the method the laboratory will use to communicate with you about this testing and what measures are taken to protect your confidentiality.

Things to consider related to undergoing genetic testing

- Difficult considerations for current or future health
- Insurance coverage issues
- Career
- Marriage
- Family building
- The need for immediate or extended family members to be tested

Some Reviews of Genetic Testing Companies

(Please note: I have no profitable disclosures to note or affiliations either personal or professional with any company mentioned in this book. The company 23andMe, discussed below, happened to be the one with which I chose to explore my own genome. Additional online options include Ancestry.com, Family Tree DNA.com, and Complete Genomics.com.)

23andMe is one of many companies doing direct-to-consumer genetics testing. It is based in Mountain View, California. For $99, 23andMe offers a saliva-based test from which is generated a "Health Overview." The Overview provides personal genomic information broken down into the following sections: health risks, inherited conditions, drug response, and inherited traits.

23andMe reports are broken into four broad and valuable categories

- **Health Risk:**, Your risk for things such as type 2 diabetes, cancers, or heart diseases
- **Inherited Conditions** (also known as **Carrier Status**): For genetically passed disease such as sickle cell anemia, Tay Sachs disease and cystic fibrosis
- **Drug Response:** How your system uniquely processes medication
- **Inherited Traits:** Eye and hair color, male pattern baldness, lactose intolerance, and cholesterol levels

More detailed technical reports are available. You can get very specific information, such as knowing whether or not you carry multiple gene variants that predispose you to disease. Additional offerings from the 23andM3 website include discussion forums, opportunities to connect with people related to you, and research of your ancestry.

A Forbes on line article features a video link of a presentation by Anne Wojcicki, co-founder and CEO of 23andme. In this clip, she elaborates on instances in which 23andme has been an enormously valuable vehicle for people to discover not only carrier status for genetically passed diseases but also drug intolerances. She spurs conversations within families about extended family health histories and presents other truly amazing research.[18]

23andMe regularly launches surveys in which thousands of people participate. At first glance it may seem a far stretch to consider this as valuable research. However, the sheer volume of people logging into the site each day provides ongoing, large samples of data collection. Solid medical research requires large and varied sample sizes of people and is typically difficult and very expensive to acquire in a conventional research setting.

For example, one example discusses involves a family with gene variant for pancreatic cancer. The family contemplated funding research to determine if a particular gene was the culprit in the cancers developing in their family members. To assist the family, 23andMe put out a survey specifically about this topic, and in 12 hours they had 12,000 surveys returned! That is a staggering response for any type of inquiry tool. As it turns out, 157 members of 23andMe carried that same gene variant. The family was able to determine that the suspected gene was in fact not the culprit causing the cancers within their family and then invested their resources in more targeted research.

Another online genetic testing site founded in 2008 is Pathway Genomics, based in San Diego, California (www.pathway.com). Its website states that it is geared toward providing physicians with "actionable genetic testing results" on insight topics, including hereditary cancers, pain medications, cardiac issues, healthy weight, carrier status and mental health.

Because I highly regard the review of genetic testing results with appropriate guidance and medical management, Pathway Genomics could be an excellent company to consider. It offers a good option for consumers who wish to submit samples through their medical doctor right from the beginning. That being said, in my clinical practice I frequently find that women desire to preview the test and the results before meeting with their medical doctor. They want to make the most of their appointment time, feel educated in the questions they pose to their practitioners, and then collaborate on the best course of action.

For those of you who would like to pursue in-depth study of your genetics through scientific papers that discuss gene mutations, I suggest looking at www.Promethease.com. Promethease is a literature retrieval system that builds you a personal DNA report based on the scientific literature cited in SNPedia along with your file of genotype (DNA) data which you provide.

Your data must first be generated from a DNA testing service such as 23andMe, FamilyTreeDNA, Ancestry.com, or Complete Genomics. You then upload it into the Promethease system. This system is perhaps one of the easiest to access and it is fascinating. It is one of the most detailed tools I have found and costs only $5 to generate a report that gathers vast amounts of scientific literature. It is available online for 45 days. My report was generated within 12 minutes; the maximum turnaround time is 20 minutes.

Promethease has solid, effective privacy practices in place such that all raw data is deleted within seconds of the reports being generated. After 45 days, reports are deleted from Promethease's system. It is easy to download your report for future reference and it is valuable to resubmit and run reports at intervals because new SNPs are discovered daily.

Science Nerd Corner

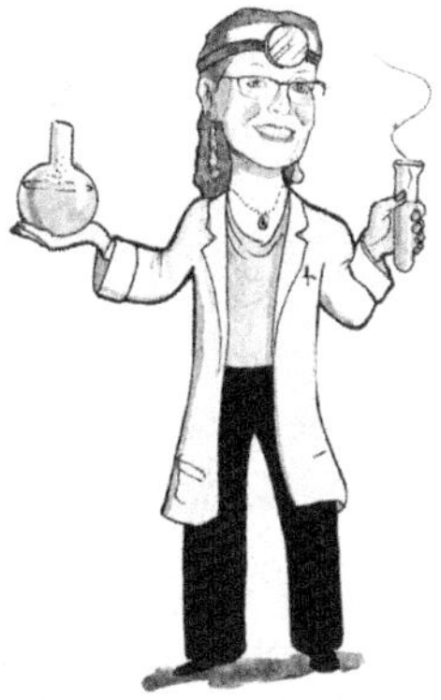

SNPs, or "snips," refer to single nucleotide polymorphisms. They are modifications in the DNA building blocks of adenine (A), thymine (T), guanine (G), and cytosine (C).

An SNP is a difference in one of the building blocks above or a difference in the order of those building blocks. Most have no significant effect on health. However, some can actually predict things like response or tolerance to drugs, risks of developing illness, or sensitivity to toxins, etc. There is great scientific interest in logging and studying SNPs in order to improve medical care.

Here are two You Tube links about Promethease. The second link is a bit older but it is valuable with respect to the detail using filters and searches within your report.

https://www.youtube.com/watch?v=QPF7IanRqok&feature=iv&src_vid=mbbRhGJhsg8&annotation_id=annotation_3779849255

https://www.youtube.com/watch?v=mbbRhGJhsg8

The Promethease Report

- Grey box items are items of interest but usually neutral with respect to health
- Green box items are "good" facts
- Red box items are "bad" or risk facts
- Order is according to magnitude, a term for gauging how important a gene is
- The UI Version 2 Interactive Report is key for in-depth research of SNPs.

Within your Promethease report you can search by topic and find out all of your SNPs that mention your topic of interest. It is possible to combine search topics, such as cancer and longevity. You will find what are called "rs numbers" pertinent to your SNPs. These are standard identification numbers set by the National Center for Biotechnology at the National Institutes of Health. If you click on an rs number, all the scientific literature collected about this position on the genome will be accessed, and links for PubMed articles will be noted if available. Newer papers are always at the bottom. You will also find exceedingly detailed information on which chromosomes and at what places on the chromosomes these mutations occur. Sorting by frequency will sort to find more rare genetic issues that pertain to you.

CHAPTER

5

THE INTERSECTION OF ACUPUNCTURE, FERTILITY & GENETICS

THE INTERSECTION OF ACUPUNCTURE, FERTILITY & GENETICS

The classics of Chinese medicine are the ancient texts from which have originated acupuncture, the use of Chinese herbs, and various nutritional and exercise practices. The classics discuss what are called the 5 Elements. The Elements are: Fire, Earth, Metal, Water and Wood. All living beings are made up of these 5 ingredients. Each of us has what is called a Constitutional Factor (C-CF), meaning that one of the 5 Elements is key for that person and will manifest mentally, physically and emotionally as strengths and also as their challenges.

{Please note that the terms "C-CF" and "constitution," are equal and interchangeable for the purposes of this book. The more common way an acupuncturist refers to constitution is "CF." However, I do not want to cause confusion with the abbreviation for cystic fibrosis, also CF, used earlier in this book. Thus for clarity and consistency, C-CF refers to "Chinese Medicine Constitution Factor" and is interchangeable with "constitution."}

Another way of understanding "constitution" is that you have a ruling element, which heavily influences your health, your well-being, what types of illnesses you might get, and how you navigate through daily life. Your C-CF influences aspects of life, such as who or what you are most comfortable with as well as conditions in which you are not. It influences to what you are drawn and also those things that make you want to run for cover. It also can predispose you to patterns of disease or illness.

At first glance, the theory seems foreign or kind of "touchy feely," but there are many valid applications of this medicine that help people handle body, mind, and spiritual stressors in life—even infertility challenges! In fact, research studies show that people with similar Chinese medicine constitutions actually have similar genetics too. One example is a 2007 study, reported in the *Journal of Alternative and Complementary Medicine,* wherein 706 healthy people were divided into groupings according to their Chinese medicine constitution. The participants' blood was genetically tested for what are called human leukocyte antigens (HLAs). HLAs are part of the immune system and are scientifically recognized as useful genetic markers to show things like autoimmune disease, predisposition to infectious diseases, hereditary diseases, and cancers. It was found that specific HLA genetic changes were shared in common by members of each constitution, as defined by traditional Chinese medicine.[19]

You may be wondering why I am presenting a discussion about 5 Element acupuncture when this book, *Baby Blueprints*, is about genetic testing. I do this because your constitution is your blueprint, just as your genetic makeup is your blueprint. My specialty, fertility acupuncture, intimately and inseparably joins with conventional medicine—I witness this connection between Chinese medicine and genetics every day.

My patients benefit from my nursing background as well as my acupuncture background. My training in both 5 Element theory diagnosis as well as traditional Chinese medicine styles of acupuncture addresses both realms: the C-CF with its gifts and challenges and the musculoskeletal body amid its gifts and challenges.

It is fascinating and gratifying that science is now illustrates this bond. A 2009 study states this very well: "…DNA may serve as a platform to integrate individual differences research across the life sciences, even including one of the most integrative and holistic medical systems inherited from East Asian tradition…"[20]

How each man copes with the male fertility factor or how each woman copes with an inability to become pregnant is impacted in large part by their uniqueness. Two people with the same medical diagnosis might have fundamentally different goals, needs, and types of acupuncture, which benefit them. One part of my job is to support patients in a highly individualized manner. Another part is to support the biophysiology of each person by treating them with acupuncture and Chinese herbs.

Understanding your fundamental constitution through pregnancy and family building can be of great value to you. An added bonus is the insight the 5 Elements can give you as parents in understanding your babies. They will enter this world with their own unique genetic and constitutional makeup, and, more often than not, it may be radically different from your own. Think about it for a moment—it is gloriously soothing to be around someone who "gets" you; you have pleasant memories of being with this person. It is painfully opposite when you feel misunderstood or pressed by someone into acting in a way that is incongruent with your natural mode.

A dear friend of mine is a Metal constitution. Metal C-CFs are often misunderstood souls. They are deeply creative and also the type of people who talk less in social situations than those with other constitutions. This is not because anything is wrong but because it is their nature to observe and experience life, not to emote or flap around. Sometimes society views Metal C-CFs as being cold or judgmental. Some people feel reluctant to be affectionate with them. The reality is that their calm, seemingly cool outside masks a party going on within them.

This friend is very successful and has a loving mate and family. One day as we were chatting about constitutions she said to me that her quite elderly mother recently said to her, "I never did understand you." I could see pain and loss in my sweet friend's eyes as she described the sting of contempt, with the inference that the mother's problem in relating to her daughter was the daughter's fault. The painful reality is likely that the mother did want to understand her daughter but didn't have the skills or insight to do this.

I think it's safe to say that no one wants to feel like an oddball. The social reality is that each constitution is typically misunderstood in some respects, and each constitution will have certain similar struggles, which tend to be recurring patterns in life. I hope this book helps you understand how to take care of yourself and your constitution and how to interact with and identify other constitutions and thus gives you valuable insight into your children and family. All 5 constitutions are gifted, needed, and amazing.

A broad understanding of constitutions can give you some tools to relate not only to your kids but also people in your family, business, and day-to-day life. It is very easy to cultivate the ability to interact with all C-CFs. Your C-CF and your genes will influence how you navigate life on all levels—physical, mental and spiritual. Your babies' C-CFs and genes will influence their lives in the same way.

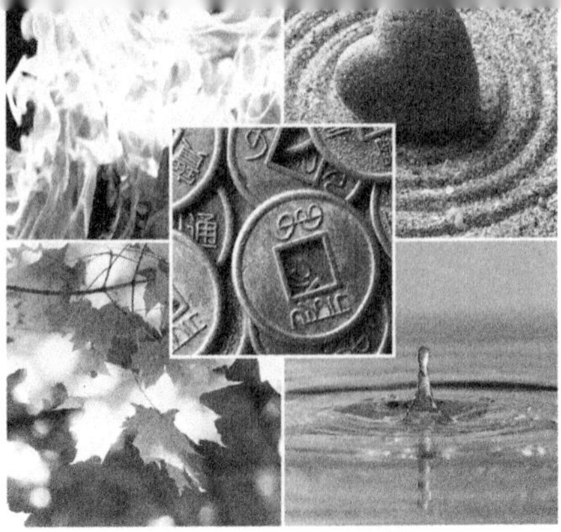

About the 5 Elements in General

A traditionally conducted 5 Element diagnosis is methodical, factual, and always respectful of the patient. An important part of it concerns observation. For example, it is striking when comparing facial complexions of a row of persons who are all Wood constitutional factors sitting next to a Water C-CF. There are even obvious ways each constitution physically moves through space. For example there are palpable differences between how a woman with a Fire constitution sits down on a chair compared to how an Earth constitution settles into a seat.

My teacher, Niki Bilton, MAc (UK), MBAcC (UK), L.Ac (MD) conducts what are called Color, Sound, Odor, Emotion (CSOE) Carnivals (http://tendingshenacupuncture.com/). These classes are comprised of practitioners or non-medical persons who take the opportunity, usually over a weekend, to learn the characteristics of each constitution and then compare and contrast people. Participants hear distinct differences in sound and cadence of each type of voice, witness how different kinds of people move, and observe how each constitution interacts with others. If you ever have an opportunity to experience a CSOE Carnival, you will find it is fun-filled and fascinating. You will certainly come away with tools that will enable you to understand and be harmonious with at least one person with whom you never previously could gel. It can also give you invaluable insight into yourself.

{The use of the word "carnival" to describe this event pertains only to the fact that on the afternoon of the final day there are designated tents for each group of constitutions—a tent designated for those with Fire constitutions, another reserved for Water C-CFs, etc. All participants have an opportunity to cycle through each tent for several minutes to observe groupings of individuals of each Element. The distinctions are remarkable, often humorous, and they ultimately facilitate an understanding of how to interact and better understand people who might be quite different from you.}

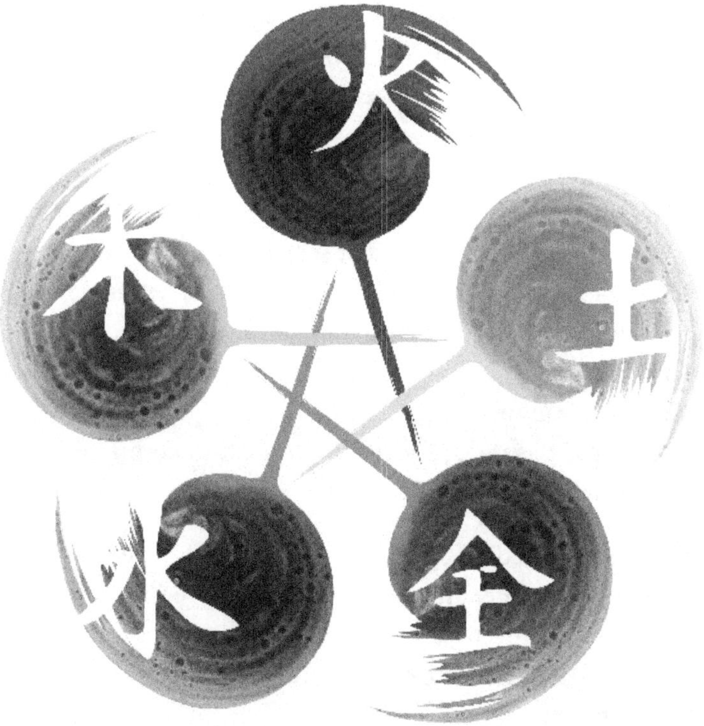

"Color," "Sound," "Odor," and "Emotion" are diagnostic terms taken from classics of Chinese medicine. It is important to remember that translations of acupuncture medical terms from classical Chinese often require precise definition and explanation just like complicated genetic terms require this. These terms may sound weird in part due to translation from ancient Chinese and in part because the diagnosis is not based upon lab tests or vital sign readings or status of X-rays or CAT scans. For example, the term "Odor" does NOT refer to stinky things and "Emotion" does NOT refer to the venting of deep dark secrets, traumas, or skeletons emerging from closets. "Odor" as a Chinese medical term refers to basic, subtle scents of each element, none of which are offensive in a healthy person. "Emotion," when used as a Chinese medical term, is often ascertained by the cadence of the voice and the specifics of how a person communicates. There are qualities such as celebration, thoughtfulness, connection, loss, vigilance and assertion associated with each of the five individual Elements.

I want to share with you some information about each of the five constitutions because it may be helpful regarding the choices you make for yourself. If this interests you, you may find value in consulting with a practitioner trained in 5 Element acupuncture. Please remember that the following is not meant for diagnosis; it is simply comparing and contrasting each Element as they present in a context of common physical complaints and fertility-related topics.

The Chinese medicine classics name the 5 Elements as Fire, Earth, Metal, Water and Wood. They also call the 5 Elements the "5 phases" because they are examples of how materials move, appear, and behave in nature. Their analysis of similar characteristics about a person tells us a great deal about their unique constitution. Listed below are some descriptions of the five Constitutional Factors.

In my practice I do address this list of fertility diagnoses with acupuncture, but please note, I am not reviewing these patterns specifically relating to constitutions mentioned in this book. The medical issues noted below can develop for any constitution depending upon a host of accompanying variables, such as heredity, environment, diet, history of accidents/injuries/surgeries/infections/toxic exposures/or illness, etc.

- Lack of ovulation
- Repeated miscarriage
- Endometriosis
- Pelvic adhesions
- Uterine fibroids/polyps
- Irregular menstrual cycles
- Painful menstrual cycles
- Heavy menstrual cycles
- PCOS
- Premature ovarian failure
- Male factor

The Fire Constitution

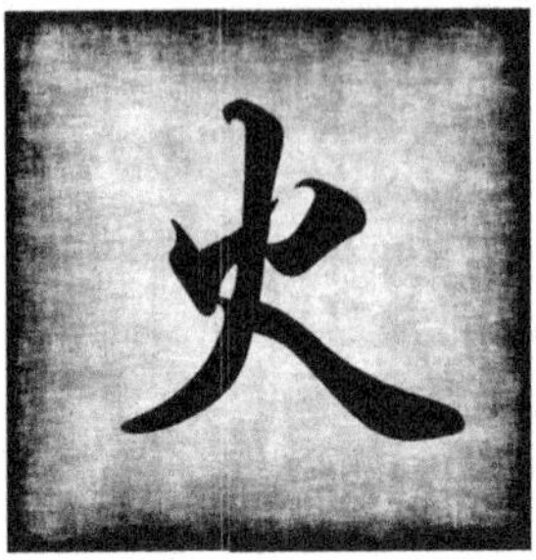

Summer is the season of the Fire Constitution, and the movement of Fire is wafting up and down like a bird gliding on winds. Think of flames rising and falling in a crackling fire. The fuel catches fire, flares, and then smolders. This is the movement of Fire. It is not possible for a fire to burn at an entirely high intensity or an only low intensity. The movement of fire naturally undulates up and down. The woman who is a Fire C-CF has an eye gaze which sparkles as it rises and falls. While chatting, he or she will look at you and then generally look away at intervals, and their eyes will seem to twinkle if something delights them. Eyebrows do a great deal bouncing around in Fire constitutions, especially if the person is telling stories and knows that they are amusing you. This is a healthy manifestation of Fire. There is no fire in the natural world, which can burn hot and roaring and not eventually burn itself out completely. There must be a fall to allow for the next rise. There must be rest after activity. People with Fire C-CF require recovery time to recharge after having fun. They are prone to over excitement and can suffer from it.

I have a distinct memory from childhood of my friend Talia's bane of existence that her younger sister would get so excited about things that she would literally faint. If the family was getting ready to board an airplane, going out trick or treating, or leaving for an amusement park, it was common for Talia's sister to temporarily pass out. The fainting would invariably cause a delay in whatever fun-filled activity was planned because her parents then needed to make sure the little sister was OK. I'm certain the sister was a Fire C-CF. I remember laughing at Talia when she would impatiently say to her sister: "Don't you dare faint this time! I do not want to have to wait around." This pattern is well-known in Chinese medicine. A typical response of Fire constitutions is the tendency toward over excitement, which flares up and temporarily wipes the person out.

Fire constitutions can be infectious flirts and insufferable gossips but not in a malicious or negative way. There is a desire to create celebration and establish a relationship and have everyone join in, for example, at a backyard barbeque or a cotillion. It's all good for the Fire C-CF as long as there is equal sharing in the social experience. The type of gathering is unimportant; it's the sharing and being together which is the goal.

Fire C-CFs can accidentally seem to verbally interrupt stories because they want to "join in." Their experience of participating in the conversation can be perceived as an interruption to the story line. This not about the Fire C-CF needing to entertain everyone. In fact, most Fire C-CFs do not feel comfortable in the limelight at all. Many a Fire constitution prefers one on one social interactions rather than giant parties. The "join in" is more accurately an invitation for equal sharing of stories, life events, and happiness. So being in social or professional situations where others are aloof, disinterested, or critical will invariably cause a Fire C-CF to retreat. All 5 Elements use humor and all 5 Elements laugh; however, it is Fire ones who most easily endear themselves to people with their natural propensity to joy. In health, they have an infectious sense of humor, which draws people in.

A Picture of the Healthy Fire Constitution

(not a complete list or to be used for diagnosis)

- Love stories and appreciate mutual sharing of stories
- Communicates with hands and gestures
- Engages easily in conversation
- Tends toward affectionate touch
- Enjoys ritual or ceremony such as celebrations and gatherings
- Can become exhausted from overdoing it in the party department
- Stop chatting only at night
- Have eyes that twinkle when something delights them
- Has contagious laughter, which reels people in
- Color=Complexion slightly reddens or flushes upward when animated
- Sound=Laugh, can have voices which tend to slightly crack while talking somewhat like crackling branches in a fireplace
- Odor=Scorched. Remember this is a Chinese translation of a medical term. All healthy constitution scents are positive and very subtle. This is classically defined as slightly floral like the first light of morning sun shining onto plants.
- Emotion=Joy/Elation

Typical complaints/patterns I see with Fire constitution fertility patients:

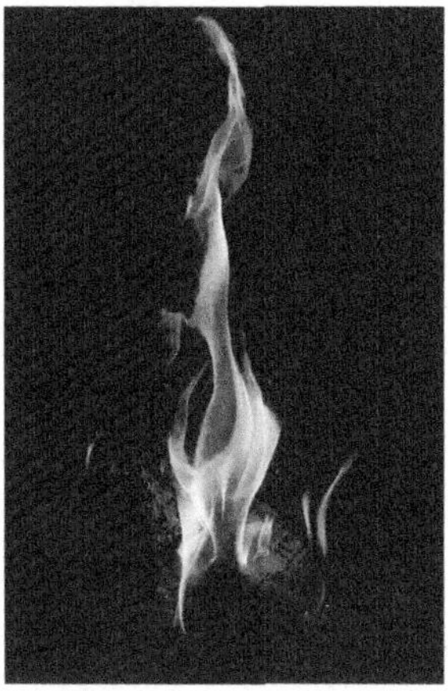

- Inability to control laughter or laughter when uncomfortable
- Sadness
- Anger
- Control issues
- Difficulty sifting and sorting information for decision--making
- Sense of feeling vulnerable in interpersonal interactions or avoiding social situations

Symptoms related (but not solely limited) to the Fire Element pathology

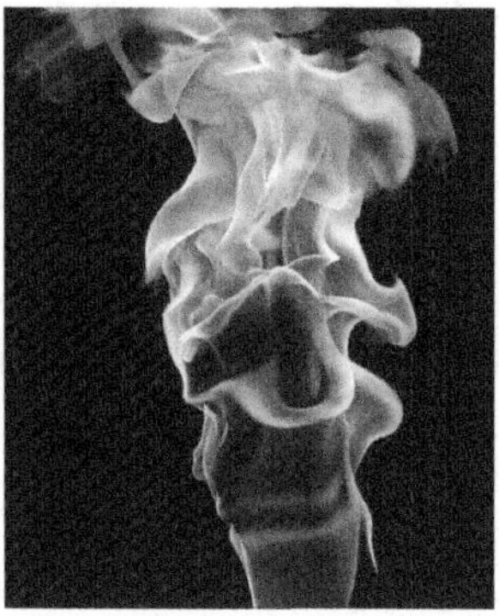

- Pale, tired, palpitations, easily sweating, shortness of breath with activity
- Anemia
- Circulation issues: cold hands or feet, issues with varicose veins
- Frequently cold, feeling chest stuffiness
- Dizziness, poor sleep, memory problems, anxiety restless, dry mouth

The Earth Constitution

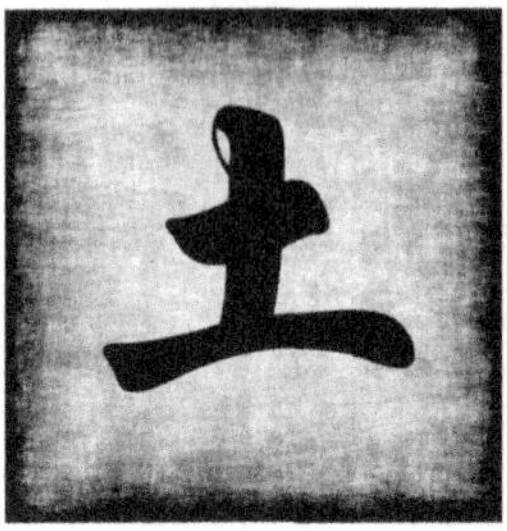

The season of the Earth element is translated as late summer or the transition between each of the four seasons. The natural movement of Earth is called "center to periphery." Earth is considered central, also known as the pivot. This is because all things must move through Earth and depend upon Earth for sustenance. For example: Fire is generated from things on the Earth, such as sticks. Metal is mined from the Earth. Wood must first grow upon the Earth before being harvested. Water springs from the depths of the Earth. All things must pass through Earth.

This movement of Earth, which is translated as center to periphery is initially rather hard to grasp. However, if for example you observe an Earth constitution woman enter a classroom you will see this movement in their gait. They will likely choose the most comfortable chair available, will settle into the seat of their choice centrally, and unpack the day's essentials from their bag. This movement illustrates center to periphery, the containment of goodies, and then the spreading about of goodies. The Chinese classics speak of Earth as safeguarding the granaries as in accumulating and sheltering food sources and then distributing those resources to support the community.

Women who are Earth constitutions want large amounts of data and information, will seek to use data and information purposefully, and are often generous in sharing it with others. They are the women in my practice who maintain detailed files of their lab work, complete with notes, inquiries, and questions. They are the students in a class who typically ask many questions. They are the friends who tell you long and detailed stories. The details are intended to give you most information possible. This is a contrast with Fire constitutions who may tell stories to entertain, create joy and encourage you to join in. The Earth C-CF is about giving you lots of data and this constitution will get easily annoyed if interrupted in their communications to you or if they experience being "cut short" in their delivery.

One of my Earth C-CF patients described a vacation she planned for her family. She was so disappointed that one of the sites on their itinerary was closed. Her children were grumbling about her being such a "control freak about needing to do every blasted thing." However, her true goal was to provide for her family so they could have the best time possible and enjoy as much as possible. Sometimes Earth constitutions' motives are incorrectly interpreted as control when they are truly altruistic. There is always an underpinning of building community—everyone getting what they need and being thoughtful.

A Picture of the Healthy Earth Constitution

(not a complete list or to be used for diagnosis)

- Seeks out and appreciates comfort
- Often is a "foodie"
- Needs to set the stage with details when sharing a story or experience
- Asks many questions
- Thoroughly seeks out information, amasses data, and readily shares it
- Focuses on all members of groups or communities in which they are part
- Is generous and thoughtful to other with resources and in spirit
- Color=Yellow
- Sound=Singing, as in the quality of voice often used in audio books for children's stories.
- Odor=Fragrant. Remember this is a Chinese translation of a medical term. All healthy constitution scents are positive and very subtle. This is classically defined as similar to the soft smell around a bouquet of flowers and will hang in the room after the person has exited.
- Emotion=Sympathy/Thoughtfulness

Typical complaints/patterns I see with Earth constitution fertility patients:

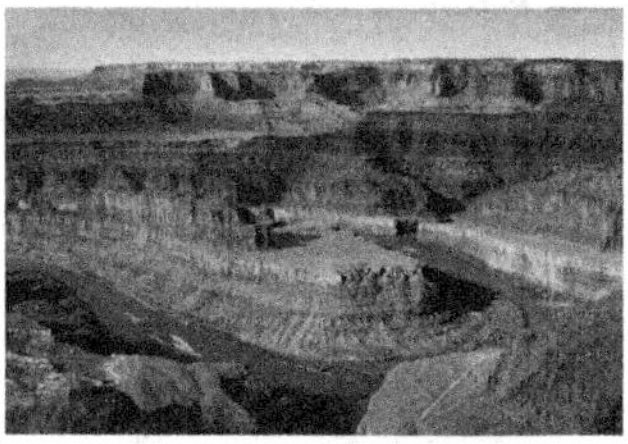

- Cramping menstrual pain during menses vs. before onset bleeding
- Menstrual cramps have a down-bearing quality
- Heavy menstrual cycles with gushing flow of blood, especially upon standing up
- Sugar cravings 2-3 days before menses
- Fatigue during menstruation
- Hemorrhoids

Symptoms related (but not solely limited) to the Earth Element pathology

- Loose stools

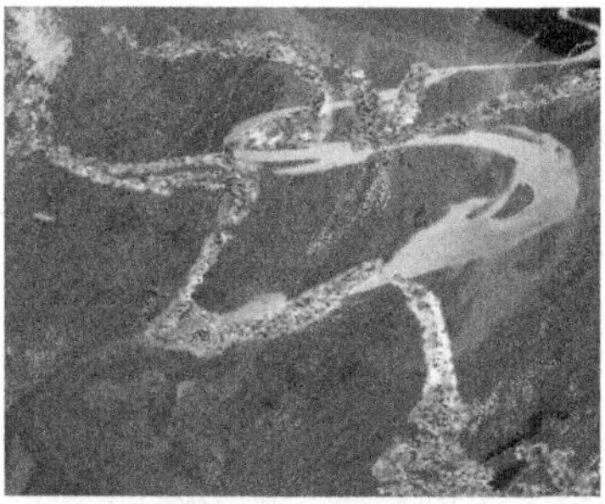

- Fatigue that improves with sitting down and propping up legs
- Fuzzy headed/dizzy
- Complaint of being cold, with feet always being the coldest
- Easily swelling feet
- Complaint of legs/all limbs feeling heavy; relieved by sitting with legs propped up
- Ruminating/over thinking
- Bad breath
- Preference for warm foods/chilled foods cause discomfort
- Increased or difficult to satiate appetite

The Metal Constitution

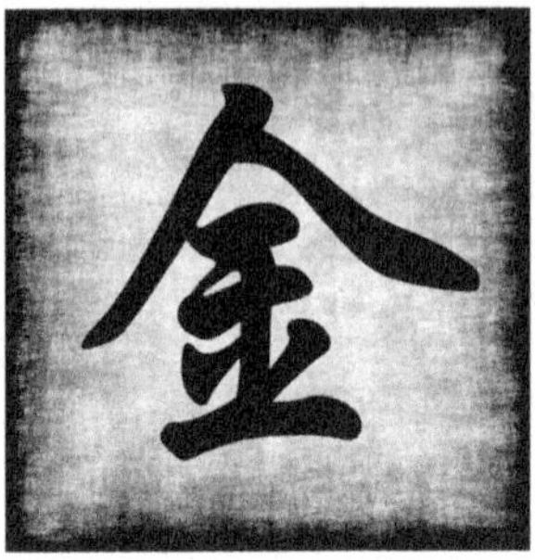

The season of the Metal constitution is autumn, and the movement of Metal is descending or moving downward. Although each of the Elements have tendencies to be misunderstood or unhelpfully pressured by society, this is especially so for women who are Metal C-CFs. In nature it is the element that can first be molded into a sword and later melted down again to become a coin. It is thus the most malleable of all of the elements. For example, if you cut a limb from a tree, there is no way to reattach it so it will again grow. If you boil away a pot of water, there is no way to recapture it, whereas metal is malleable, changeable, and actually the most amenable of the 5 Elements.

Opposite of Fire constitutions, Metal C-CFs do not talk a lot, especially when in large social situations. This is not because they are shy or unhappy; they tend to enjoy the experience of events but they do not need to verbally emote. Being pressed into chattiness is exhausting and not helpful for Metal constitutions. A woman who is a Metal constitution is not fidgety. The classics describe Metal as "inert," which means very still and composed. However, the inner world is filled with creativity and activity. We call this "Yin on the exterior, Yang on the interior" or, as a teacher of mine likes to describe it, stillness on the outside, rock and roll blaring on the inside.

Metal C-CFs tend to have a piercing gaze, which can seem to look through you. The laser beam gaze can be misinterpreted as being critical when in fact Metal C-CFs are the least judgmental of all of the constitutions. Metal is highly observant and pays great attention to detail with an appreciation of expertise. Two of my Metal patients excel in martial arts and fencing; they see physical patterns quickly and can assess situations with natural skill.

Metal constitutions are quite at ease in nature and very much enjoy and relate to animals. They experience and connect to the world around them rather than intellectually think about it or express it verbally. They experience what is called connection and loss in life or what the Chinese classics translate as grief. An example might be their intense appreciation of the flowering tree followed by the sense of loss when the necessity autumn arrives and the leaves fall.

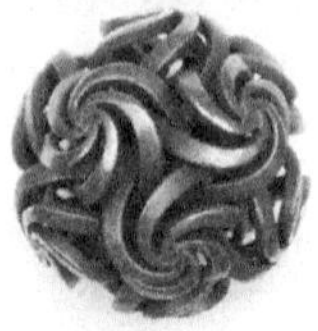

A Picture of the Healthy Metal Constitution
(not a complete list or to be used for diagnosis)

- Usually thin body type
- Cadence of the voice has mainly downward deflection, especially at the end of sentences
- Dry sense of humor
- An appreciation for sarcasm
- Stillness on the outside intense creativity on the inside
- Fascination/appreciation of textures and smells—for example, the little girl who is more fascinated with examining the jar of bugs in her pocket as opposed to other toys
- Operates on instinct and intimately connected with their surroundings
- Strong sense of justice
- Precise, i.e., in handwriting, verbal expression, etc.
- Color=White, like talcum powder lightly coating the skin
- Sound=Weep, as in sentences deflecting downward.
- Odor=Rotten. Remember this is a Chinese translation of a medical term. All healthy constitution scents are positive and very subtle. This is similar to the smell of B vitamins.
- Emotion=Grief/Connection & Loss

Typical complaints/patterns of Metal constitution fertility patients:

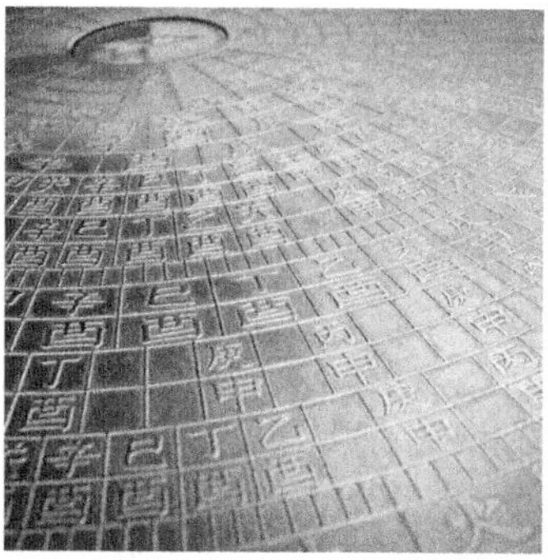

- Sense of alienation
- Difficulty gaining weight
- Constipation
- Respiratory issues, i.e., asthma, bronchitis
- Skin issues, i.e., psoriasis, eczema
- Scanty or missed menstrual cycles

Symptoms related (but not solely limited) to the Metal Element pathology

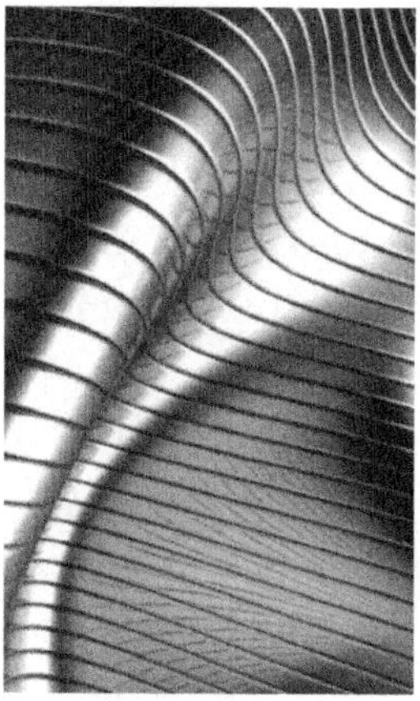

- Problems with or changes in sense of smell
- Difficulties with voice or vocal chords
- Complaint of coldness in the upper extremities
- Frequent colds or flus, migraines, missed or light menses

The Water Constitution

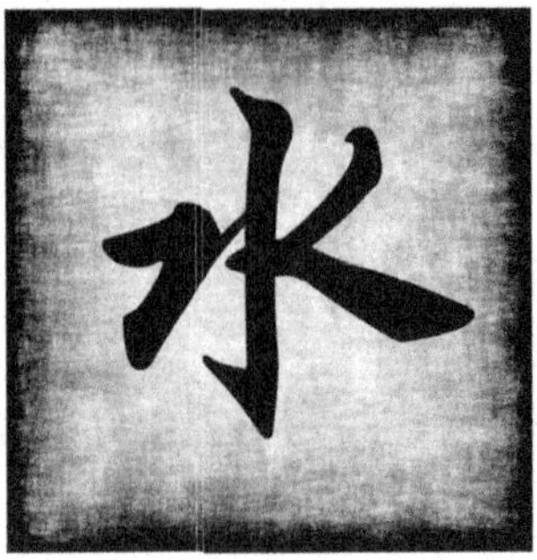

The season of the Water element is winter, and the movement is a combination of stillness and motion ultimately moving forward, just like water in nature. If you are sitting next to a lake, the surface may be calm and mostly still, but there will always be some level of motion, if only in the depths. Water constitutions are what my teacher likes to describe as "ready, ready, just in case." This is the woman who immediately springs into action if a person next to her keels over from a heart attack, if a fire breaks out in her office, or if she arrives at her parked car to find a flat tire. Healthy Water constitutions know what to do in the right moment, just like water rushing out of the newly released gates of a dam or a Harley Davidson shifting from idling to open throttle. Movement is imperative for Water constitutions. Being told they need "to do less" or "take on less" is highly annoying to them because they thrive amid activity, drama, and getting things done.

Water constitutions are known as vigilant in that they have a keen awareness of their surroundings. They will, for example, intuitively remember where all the exits are while at a large convention or will be able point out potentially dangerous surrounding before accidents occur. The classics say that the virtue of the Water C-CF is wisdom, which is the progressive accumulation of knowing how to accomplish tasks. Sometimes Water constitutions, like Wood constitutions, intimidate people. Whereas Wood can do so with its natural assertion, Water inadvertently does this owing to the natural depths of power and not being concerned with criticism or opposition.

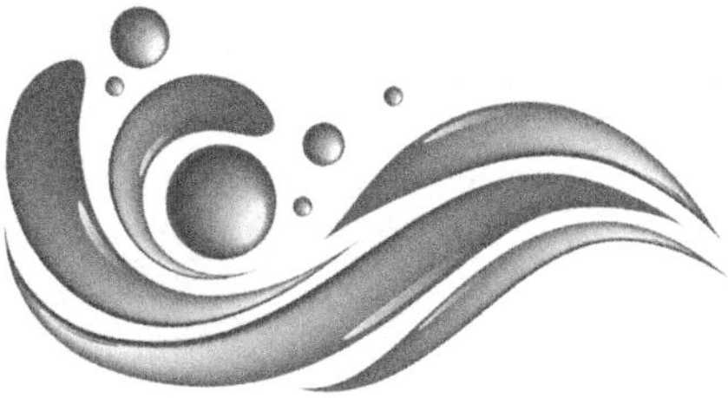

A Picture of the Healthy Water Constitution
(not a complete list or to be used for diagnosis)

- Often is louder than other Elements
- Has a more substantial physical build
- Loves to be busy
- Less inclined to take information at face value without exploration of the subject themselves.
- Eager to press forward with tasks/challenges
- Has considerable endurance for example working long hours or with physical tasks
- Their nature is compared to run away trains or crashing waves as in "get out of the way or get bowled over."
- Color=Blue/Black
- Sound=Groan
- Odor=Putrid. Remember this is a Chinese translation of a medical term. All healthy constitution scents are positive and very subtle. This is like the scent of the beach.
- Emotion=Fear/Vigilance

Typical complaints/patterns I see with Water constitution fertility patients:

- Exhaustion that improves most by lying flat on the floor

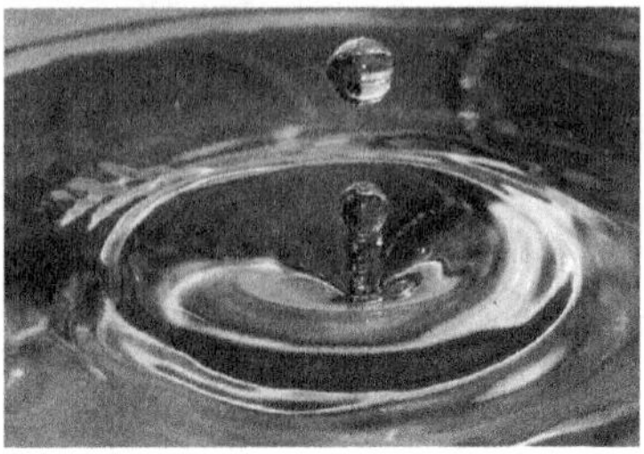

- Anxiety
- Poor sleep
- More issues with ovulation
- Recurrent miscarriage

Symptoms related (but not solely limited) to the Water Element pathology

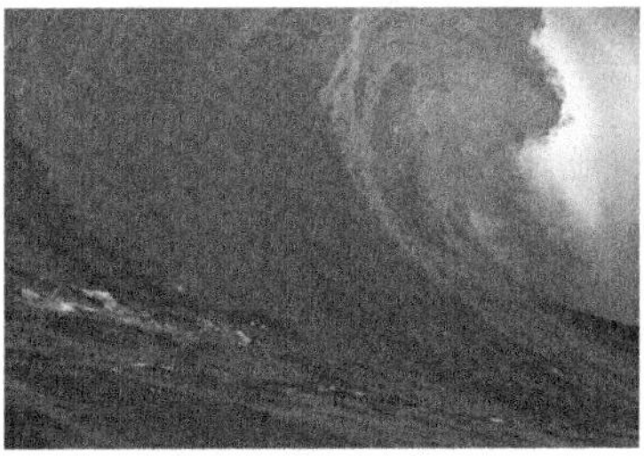

- Tendency to sprained ankles
- Complaints related to ears, teeth or hair.
- Asthma
- Tinnitus
- Swelling of the lower limbs or lower body

The Wood Constitution

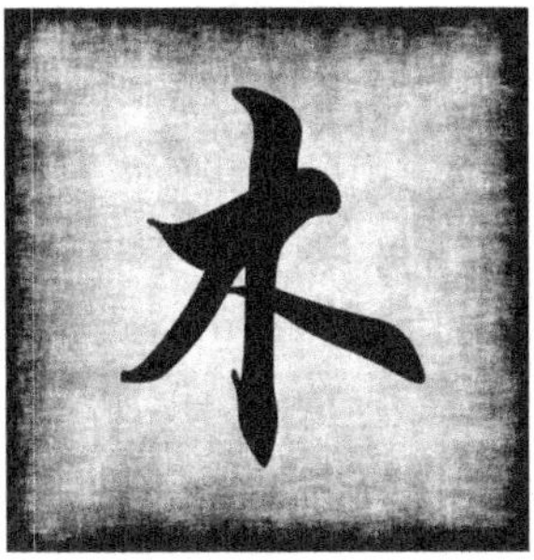

The season of the Wood element is spring and the natural movement of Wood associates with a surging up and out motion like a growing tree or a sprouting bud. This is different than the rise and fall of Fire, which slowly wafts or undulates up and down. The sound of the voice is like shouting—think of rooting for your team at a sporting event. Sports fans yell—it's fast, forceful and effective. People yell in short sentences and communicate information efficiently. They push out each syllable. The voice of the Wood C-CF is not like the Fire Constitution chatting and not like the silence of Metal constitution observing and listening. The cadence of the Wood voice is a short, staccato string of words that you might be able to shout before running out of lung power. That is not to say Wood C-CFs go about shouting or are angry people. It is more about the quality of those short, clipped sentences.

Wood constitutions often love sports or any activity involving the back and forth with a worthy, clever opponent. It's not about winning for themselves, it is about win-win for everyone. One of my Wood constitution clients is a litigation attorney. He is never contentious or aggressive in day-to-day activities, and in all the years I've known him I've never seen him raise his voice, yet he absolutely delights in the debate and the argument of law. He loves to win and loves to win for his clients. This is a healthy manifestation of Wood, which is all about benevolence, planning and well wishing.

In Chinese medicine the Wood constitution is regarded as the Element with the Grand Plan.

Of all of the 5 Elements, Wood is the best at assessing circumstances and creating successful, executable plans. Frustration creeps in for Wood C-CFs when people surrounding them do not rise to challenges or when plans are poorly constructed and do not create a win-win for all parties.

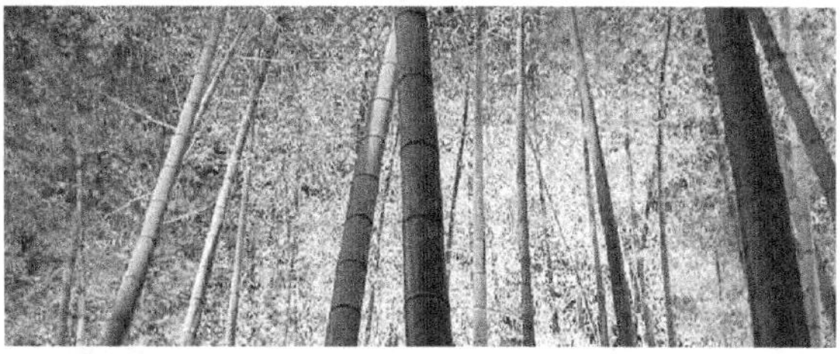

A Picture of the Healthy Wood Constitution
(not a complete list or to be used for diagnosis)

- Are most often "right" in planning situations
- Are expert in executing tasks but often question themselves because they are always striving for the best plan
- Love to play games, work puzzles, and banter back and forth in debates
- May be perceived as impatient or deflated with life obstacles in their life path
- Are no-nonsense/low drama personalities who sometime come across as intimidating due to their natural assertion
- Color=Green
- Sound=Shout
- Odor=Rancid. (Remember this is a Chinese translation of a medical term. All healthy constitution scents are positive and very subtle. This is similar to the smell of sap from green tree branches or the smell of berry bush vines before the berries ripen.)
- Emotion=Anger/Assertion (The correct understanding is Assertion or the force necessary to execute tasks. This is like a flower pushing up through a crack in the sidewalk. The flower is unlikely to be angry about it. It simply is the force necessary to be able to bloom and grow.)

Typical complaints or patterns I see with Wood constitution fertility patients:

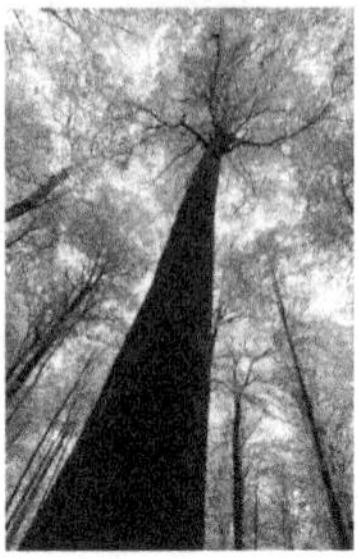

- Lack of menstruation or scanty menstruation
- Dark, black clots in menstrual flow
- Very dry eyes/frequent use of eye drops
- Irritability/frustration
- Feel markedly better if in bed before 10PM at night
- PMS worse the week leading up to menses

Symptoms related (but not solely limited) to the Wood Element pathology

- Numbness or stiffness of the arms and legs, blurred vision, dizziness, headaches, sleep walking, restless leg syndrome, muscle cramps, twitching muscles extremely pale complexion, dry/brittle/breaking nails sense of distention in flanks or between the ribs.
- Episodes of diarrhea
- Episodes of hiccups or belching
- More pronounced "growing pains" during childhood especially in the arms and legs
- Sleepwalking

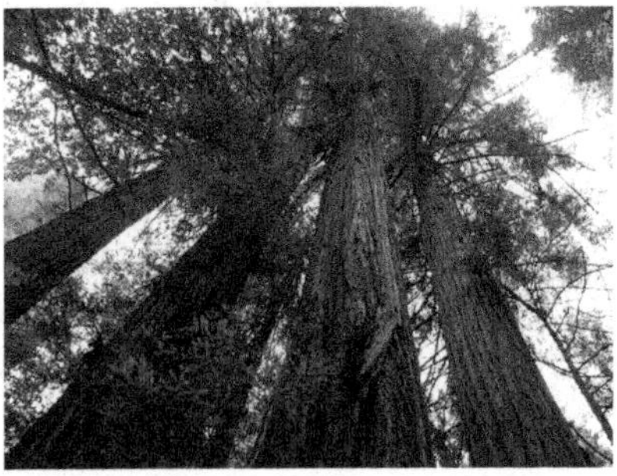

CHAPTER

6

GENETIC COUNSELING—WHY?

GENETIC COUNSELING—WHY?

A genetics counselor is highly trained to not only educate you on what tests to consider but also to educate you about the reliability of any tests you pursue. It is good to remember that there are limitations for all tests—few of them are regarded as absolutely infallible. There can be false positives as well as false negatives for many tests, and an experienced counselor can review all of those specifics with you. If you know the limitations of the tests, you'll be better prepared to review and consider the results as well as think about further testing if necessary. You will also learn about the panels recommended to be most useful to you based upon your unique family history. It may also surprise you to know that genetics counseling is frequently covered under many insurance policies.

Here is one example of testing reliability, which has to do with cystic fibrosis (CF) and the CTFR gene, which causes the disease. More than 1,000 different types of mutations have been discovered on CTFR gene, all of which produce CF. However, some of the less common types do not scar the pancreas as much as others do. Because the testing would be cost prohibitive to check for 1,000+ variants of the CTFR gene, carrier tests are typically checking for the 23 most common CTFR genetic mutations.

This brings us back to an example of test reliability. Usual CF testing will pick up about 90% of carriers. This means that 10% of the time it might be presumed that parents are not carriers but in fact are. In this situation, there is a possibility of a child with CF being born to a couple despite negative test results.

In addition to expertise in determining which types of genetics tests are needed, genetic counselors also will investigate your family history with you. At first glance, this may seem like an easy or straight forward task. However, there commonly are risk factors or indicators that the average person may not note when reviewing their family health history. You can actually begin gathering information on your family history now and below are some on-line tools.

Charles Eng, Director of the Cleveland Clinic's Genomic Medicine Institute is quoted here: "Family history is a major tool for gauging genetic risk of disease. It's a wonderful, inexpensive quick snapshot of genes and environment. Family history is the sum total of what you inherit and what you are exposed to. Once you identify someone at high risk, you can proceed to the next stage of evaluation by genetics professionals, and testing can begin if a gene is known."[21]

Tips on how to begin your family history

- List diseases your blood relatives have had (including parents, siblings, half-siblings, aunts, uncles and cousins)
- How old were these individuals at the time a disease started?
- For deceased family members, what was the cause of death?
- How old were individuals at the time of death?
- Did the deceased relatives have risk factors such as smoking, obesity, etc.?

Do you want to get started on a family history right now? If so, you can immediately begin to collect and document information for your own family history using these two online resources:

- The United States surgeon general offers a free online tool called My Family Health Portrait. Please see http://www.hhs.gov/familyhistory/portrait/ This tool allows you create a document that is organized for easily presenting information to your MD. It also allows for updating information over time, sharing it with family members or printing it out. It is available in both Spanish and English.
- The March of Dimes family history tool is available at: http://www.marchofdimes.org/materials/family-health-history-form.pdf

Within my acupuncture practice I often treat stress and anxiety reduction for clients who are considering genetic tests while looking at risk statistics. Sometimes numbers give comfort, other times not so much. It is key to remember that when you weigh facts, look at the big picture and when doing so, look at it with people who are educated in the field of genetic testing. This will give you a more informed space versus a focus on any single percentage. While part of my role is to calm the spirit, genetics counselors are trained to conduct a thorough family history, recommend tests, be supports for the seriousness of decision-making, and ultimately help you as the patient navigate complex topics.

Genetic counselor Amy Vance was kind enough to meet with me and share information about her specialty as well as her substantial clinical background and experience. Please also see her website at: http://www.bayareagc.com/BAGC/home.html.

Karen Reynolds, LAc, MS, RN
Please tell me about your background.

Amy Vance, MS, LCGC
I have a BA in zoology and completed the pre-med curriculum from Miami University. I have a master's in genetic counseling and graduated in 1991. I am also board certified by the American Board of Genetic Counseling and licensed by the State of California. Licensure for genetic counselors is relatively new and is not available in all states yet.

Karen Reynolds, LAc, MS, RN
Can you elaborate on the benefits of consulting with a genetic counselor?

Amy Vance, MS, LCGC
The major benefits are to gather information about family history and assess any possible risk to pregnancy. These are discussed, and testing can be offered *before* pregnancy because it opens a lot of options. If both individuals carry, for example, a recessive gene for the same condition, they can consider embryo screening if the couple is doing IVF. It offers people an option to avoid finding out stressful information during pregnancy, when there are fewer options.

Karen Reynolds, LAc, MS, RN
What are some pros or cons about screening prior to pregnancy?

Amy Vance, MS, LCGC
Even basic carrier screening during pregnancy is hard, because waiting for any type of test result is very stressful. If it

is an option, it is better to do the testing when not pregnant because it is less waiting, wondering and worrying. It gives more of a footing for decision- making.

Karen Reynolds, LAc, MS, RN
For women who are trying to conceive, what does genetic counseling entail and what are the most typical genetic tests offered?

Amy Vance, MS, LCGC
First, a Family Health Risk Assessment is made for three generations of family history. It is then discussed and analyzed. For most people, this screening tool in and of itself clarifies individual medical issues.

In addition to the risk assessment, genetic screening for Society recommended diseases can be offered. The American Congress of Obstetricians and Gynecologists (ACOG), the American Society for Reproductive Medicine (ASRM), and the American College of Medical Genetics (ACMG) have certain guidelines for carrier screening.

I don't do larger (non-society based) genetic testing panels. The large extended screening panels typically screen for over 50-100 variants, which increases the number of people who test positive significantly. Additionally, typically these panels don't screen for all mutations for each condition. So if you are "negative," you are only "negative" for certain mutations on the panel. I advocate offering a test in the context of genetic counseling and appropriate follow up, providing knowledge of testing limitations, and giving support if a test is positive.

People can get incorrect information or misinformation in the absence of proper support and that can do potential harm.

Karen Reynolds, LAc, MS, RN
What are the inadequacies you see in current pregnancy related genetic testing?

Amy Vance, MS, LCGC
In the prenatal setting, anyone over 35 at the time of delivery in the state of California is referred to genetic counselor. However, most OBs do not refer women under the age of 35 years for preconception genetic counseling.

It is also standard that most OB's do not see patient until week 8 of pregnancy, which is because there is a high miscarriage risk in the first 8 weeks.

Another point many consumers do not understand is that most of the time, genetic counseling is covered by insurance, and you can meet with a genetic counseling before becoming pregnant.

Genetic counseling can be thought of as a way to receive information about options during pregnancy, including family history screening, genetic testing and screening including blood testing, prenatal diagnosis, and ultrasound. Genetic testing is optional and the genetic counselor can help you understand what information is available and how it can help inform you during your pregnancy.

Karen Reynolds, LAc, MS, RN
It sounds as though there are needs in the realm of the egg donor population for genetic counseling as well then?

Amy Vance, MS, LCGC
Donors who are asked to consent to genetic testing deserve informed consent about what the testing is and what the test

results mean. They deserve to be provided genetic counseling for positive test results. Many times this does not occur. There are no specific regulations or requirements regarding provision of genetic counseling in this situation.

One idea I had was charging an extra $50 for genetic counseling for each donor. The fee is nominal and would be pooled and used for counseling donors and educating intended parents. Yes, it would cost everyone a bit more, however, at least there would not be a penalty for the donor with a positive test result.

An organization called SEEDS is currently working with donor agencies, genetic counselors, attorneys to try to achieve guidelines for certain processes related to egg donation, including genetic counseling and testing. ASRM currently does not address these specific issues.

Karen Reynolds, LAc, MS, RN
Thank you, Amy for sharing your time and expertise. For further information, please see Amy's Bay Area Genetic Counseling website at: www.bayareagc.com

CHAPTER

7

THE MOST MODERN GENETICS WITH IVF

THE MOST MODERN GENETICS WITH IVF

Reproductive challenges are all too common these days. You may know someone struggling with getting pregnant or perhaps you are struggling with this yourself. In the last ten years, the genetic testing possibilities have exploded, offering couples tools for dramatically increasing success in becoming pregnant and carrying a healthy, happy baby to term.

For the purposes of pre-implantation genetic diagnosis (within an assisted reproductive or IVF setting) and/or prenatal genomic screening (once a pregnancy is under way) testing is done to detect aneuploidy. This term refers to either extra or missing chromosomes, which will impact health. Testing offers immense benefits on multiple levels. First, it allows for the possibility within a reproductive medicine setting to only transfer embryos that have the healthy compliment of chromosomes. Since the likelihood of chromosomal abnormality rises markedly with maternal age, this can avoid transfers of embryos which are destined not to be viable, avoids the heart break and expense of failed cycles, and avoids delayed interventions which a couple may face later in a pregnancy.

A 2013 article published in *Fertility and Sterility cited that the Centers of Disease Control* noted that less than 19% of transferred embryos result in a viable baby. This same clinical trial showed an 84.7% delivery rate for the group, which had comprehensive chromosome screening as compared with the non-tested group, which had a 67.5% delivery rate.[22] To give you a sense of likelihood of chromosomal abnormalities in embryos, I'll share with you results of another multicenter study. This very large study, 2009-13, looked at data from 956 embryos (blastocysts). Of the women who participated, the mean age was 37.8 years. The overall rate of embryos with chromosomal abnormalities was 55.5%, meaning that slightly more than half of all possible embryos were not genetically destined to produce healthy babies. This obviously reflects a profound value on many levels to genetic testing within the reproductive medicine setting.[23]

Second, for future generations, use of comprehensive chromosome screening can prevent the spread of genetic disease within a family line. Third, it offers invaluable information for couples, which might be the possibility of not carrying a pregnancy to term knowing that a severe genetic disorder has occurred or to plan for the arrival for special needs child. It is all highly personal. One of my goals in producing this book is to provide information so that you can make the most informed and educated decisions, which are right for you and your family.

Next is an interview with Dr. Christo Zouves of the Zouves Fertility Center in Foster City, California. Dr. Zouves kindly shared his time with me and gave me a tour of his state of the art facility. Zouves Fertility Center opened its doors in 1999 as the first IVF laboratory in the country to become College of American Pathologists (CAP) accredited in molecular pathology. Dr Zouves elaborates about the benefits of on-site genetic testing of embryos.

Karen Reynolds, LAc, MS, RN:
Thank you, Dr. Zouves, for meeting with me to do this interview. It is my goal to provide people with understandable, up-to-date information, which they then can use to make educated decisions about their fertility and family building. You are one of the few

reproductive endocrinologists consistently using genetic testing and even doing it on-site in your own accredited laboratory. Can you give me some background about how you chose this technology and path?

Dr. Christo Zouves: The Human Genome Project was first discussed by the U.S. government in 1984 and work on the project was started in 1990 under the auspices of the NIH with private companies like Celera working in parallel starting in 1998. Valuable work was also done in France and Japan culminating in the announcement in 2003 that the human genome had essentially been mapped. As the gene sequence of individual genes causing inherited disease became known, it became possible to identify this gene in the blood of individuals who were carrying the gene, and, by extension, we became able to test embryos before implanting them back into the uterus through assisted reproduction.

As a reproductive endocrinologist doing IVF since 1984, the ability to identify single genes that cause a specific disease as well as the ability to check on chromosomal numbers allowed us to approach the individual embryo with a view to removing a cell and testing that cell for the single gene disorder or to confirm a normal number of chromosomes. Initially, the biopsy was performed on day three, removing a single cell from an embryo containing eight cells, but in the last three years, we have moved to doing the biopsy on day 5 or 6, where approximately five cells are removed from an embryo containing approximately 150 cells.

The technology is now available to test those cells for single gene disorders as well as chromosomal numbers through the development of the technique called comprehensive chromosomal screening (CCS).

CCS is a procedure that allows us to look for the presence of aneuploidy* like Down syndrome or other trisomies as well as abnormalities in the sex chromosomes like Turner's syndrome, Klinefelter syndrome, or single gene disorders, such as those associated with cystic fibrosis (CF), Tay Sachs (TS), or spinal muscular atrophy (SMA). One of the most amazing benefits of this testing is that it can remove a bad gene from a family line forever and identify an embryo which could result in an abnormal baby.

Karen Reynolds, LAc, MS, RN:
Can you describe some of the specific benefits or strengths of using genetic testing?

Dr. Christo Zouves: The ability to identify normal embryos allows us now to transfer one single normal embryo to the uterus after IVF, thereby almost eliminating the risk of multiple pregnancy and decreasing the risk of miscarriage to less than 10% while maintaining a pregnancy rate of almost 70% per normal embryo transferred. The ability to identify the single gene disorders also allows us to prevent the birth of individuals with very debilitating diseases many of which are lethal.

At the present time, the platform that we use is the Comparative Genomic Hybridization but by January 2015, next-generation sequencing (NGS) will become clinically available, allowing us to do the analysis sooner and also to allow exploration of risk forecasting for disease

We are the only reproductive laboratory in the U.S. with a CAP {College of American Pathologists} accredited laboratory for doing comprehensive chromosomal screening on-site. After the cells are removed from the embryo at the blastocyst stage, the embryo is individually vitrified and the cells are sent to our own CCS laboratory at Zouves Fertility Center. Cells removed on day 5 or 6 can be analyzed for the following abnormalities:

1. Identification of aneuploidy
2. Identification of disorders stemming from a single gene mutation
3. Identification of balanced translocations

As a fertility specialist, these three areas of testing are all important, but more than 90% of testing revolves around excluding abnormal numbers of chromosomes or aneuploidy. Single gene disorders are less common, but now that the gene sequence of more than 2000 diseases is known, we should be looking for more of these diseases in embryos in the future.

Balanced translocation is quite uncommon. It involves individual genetic material moving from one chromosome to another. Individuals with a balanced translocation are normal; however, when their bodies make eggs or sperm, the resulting gamete may become unbalanced, and this could produce an embryo that miscarries or a baby with severe congenital abnormalities A person who carries a balanced translocation may produce very few normal embryos and this makes the CCS testing especially helpful to select normal embryos for transfer.

By January 2015, we will be using next-generation sequencing (NGS) in our program. NGS is a technique that uses whole genome amplification (WGA) by polymerase chain reaction followed by DNA Library generation and sequencing by synthesis on the MiSeq platform

With NGS, we will be able to get an analysis more quickly and look at very specific areas of testing and identification.

There will also be the ability to do risk forecasting for disease with genetic sequencing and thereby show predispositions to diseases in a new way. With gene sequencing, there is the availability to test the peripheral blood of a pregnant woman and isolate fetal DNA for analysis. This noninvasive prenatal testing (NIPT) will all but eliminate the need for amniocentesis

Karen Reynolds, LAc, MS, RN:
Do you encourage women to get the conventional genetic testing at 10 weeks of pregnancy even if they have had CCS associated with their IVF cycles?

Dr. Christo Zouves: Yes, we recommend it. For us it is confirmation that the embryo analysis is correct given that the CCS technology gives an accuracy of 99.5%. Additionally it is non-invasive to the fetus and not expensive. It also means that there is less need for CVS {chorionic villus sampling} or amniocentesis.

Karen Reynolds, LAc, MS, RN:
Your center reflects a very high rate of success. Do you attribute this to the genetic testing?

Dr. Christo Zouves: Yes, please see the enclosed slides. Once you identify a normal embryo, it has the same chance of making a normal baby whether the woman is 35 years old, 40 years old or 45 years old. The challenge however is to identify a normal embryo given that by age 45, less than 5% of embryos are normal. However once we do find a normal embryo the patient will have a 70% chance of carrying to term. This is similar for a 35-year-old or a 40-year-old woman. This gives further support to the genetic testing we do. We can avoid failed cycles by not transferring embryos, which are not genetically viable, and we can decrease the rate of miscarriage to less than 10%.

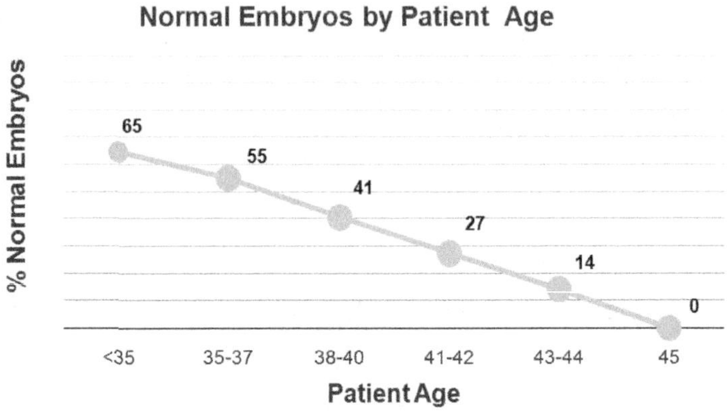

Of 1,500 embryos analyzed last year we found that 65% of blastocysts are normal for a woman under 35 years old, 41% of blastocysts are normal for a 40 year old woman, and less than 5% of blastocysts are normal for a 45-year-old woman. That is why it is so difficult to get a baby for someone whose eggs have already turned 45 without resorting to a donor egg.

Karen Reynolds, LAc, MS, RN:
Why do some IVF programs not recommend CCS?

Dr. Christo Zouves: One of their arguments against CCS is risk of damage to the blastocyst. However, the reality is that the risk is only one in every 1, 000 biopsied blastocytes. We do the biopsy on day 5 when the blastocyte is made up of roughly 150 cells. We take between 5-7 cells. Most good IVF programs are no longer doing single cell day 3 biopsy anymore because you get roughly 5 times the DNA with a 5-cell biopsy on day 5 as opposed to a single cell removed on day

3. Embryos on day 3 are much more likely to be mosaic and growing the embryos to day five cuts the risk of an embryo being mosaic dramatically.

Karen Reynolds, LAc, MS, RN:
I find often with my patients there is such an intense desire for pregnancy that women opt for transfer of multiple embryos, despite what are grave risks with multiples both with pregnancy, birth and ongoing health concerns. What are your current thoughts on transferring of multiple embryos and does your facility often transfer multiple embryos?

Dr. Christo Zouves: We do sometimes transfer more than one embryo, if, for example, someone elects not to do genetic testing. Or we may put in two embryos if a woman is over 40 years old and she has not done genetic testing. It is important to remember that for a 40-year-old woman, there is a 40% chance of an embryo being normal; so in those instances it can make sense to put in more than one. However, our current statistics show that we put in an average of 1.3 embryos per transfer for those people who do genetic testing. We also do frozen embryo transfers instead of transferring the embryos fresh when the woman has just been stimulated with fertility medication. By having a woman return a month or so later for transfer during natural ovulation, the body is more receptive and the pregnancy runs more smoothly.

Natural Cycle FET with CCS

October 2012 – September 2014

	<35	35 – 37	38 – 40	41 – 42	>42
Number of Transfers	28	39	48	21	8
Clinical Pregnancy Rate	68%	72%	60%	57%	50%
Implantation Rate	66%	66%	56%	63%	50%
Average Number of Embryos Transferred	1.17	1.23	1.29	1.28	1.25

Karen Reynolds, LA., MS, RN:
It is my clinical experience that initially the decision to reduce seems like a feasible one. Then when faced with reduction, its risks, heart breaks and worries that in fact it is never an easy decision or process.

Dr. Christo Zouves: Doing a selective reduction is a very difficult decision and it is much better to identify which embryos are normal and transfer one normal embryo at a time.

Karen Reynolds, LAc, MS, RN:
Can you please describe your facility's process for genetic counseling?

Dr. Christo Zouves: The starting point has to be with everybody completing the same assessments. Here in our office, a genetic risk assessment is mandatory. Each patient must speak with genetic counselor, Amy Vance. If you set up a screening processing, I think it is really important that all patients are evaluated by the same tools in the same way, so that nothing gets missed. Our aim is to have healthy patients and to produce healthy babies. We do test for 19 single gene disorders through a panel performed by Good Start Genetics. We test both the egg and the sperm providers.

Diet, nutrition, and supplementation re key and so is counseling around genetic risk assessment. Most people do not sit down and consider three generations of genetic risk from both sides of the family. We had one 38-year-old patient who didn't realize she had a strong family history for risk of colon cancer. We insisted that she have a colonoscopy, and it turned out she already had a developing cancer. The genetic risk assessment is to check to be sure that there are no family tendencies, which can be future risks for the woman or subsequently the child.

We very much espouse a holistic approach to IVF. Doing IVF is like training for a triathlon. You must train the mind, spirit, and body. I support and recommend acupuncture, though some people can be needle phobic. We strongly recommend exercise, yoga, and meditation. Research has shown that meditation lengthens telomeres on the chromosomes. We also stress the value of eating an organic, gluten free diet and we supply a list of supplements. For all patients we recommend a full range of supplements including CoQ10, Omega 3 fish oils, vitamin D, high dose folic acid, and high dose multi-vitamins.

Karen Reynolds, LAc, MS, RN:
With what genetic companies does Zouves Fertility Center work?

Dr. Christo Zouves: We partner with Good Start Genetics (GSG) and we use a panel, which includes ruling out genetically inherited diseases, such as thalassemia, cystic fibrosis, spinal muscular atrophy, fragile X syndrome. This allows us to look for problematic single gene presentations in the patient and then ultimately helps us find normal embryos.

Karen Reynolds, LAc, MS, RN:
Historically, it was presumed slower growth and development reflected compromised quality of the blastocyst. Now we are seeing that that embryologists will opt to cryopreserve euploid embryos even if they have demonstrated marginal morphologic quality. Are you clinically seeing that even slower developing blastocytes or ones of lower morphologic rating are resulting in pregnancies and babies?

Dr. Christo Zouves: I think it's true that embryos, which hit landmark developmental markers within specific time frames are more likely to be normal. The gold standard is still to do CCS. Ideally, an embryo needs to be a blastocyst on day 5, which will have an edge on a blastocyst that does not meet the landmark development markers by that time. We have also use continuous videography, which allows us to assess which blastocysts hit these landmarks first. Continuous videography does not differentiate normal from abnormal and we now use exclusively CCS to identify the single embryo for transfer.

Karen Reynolds, LAc, MS, RN:
Since you are one of the few reproductive endocrinologists standardly incorporating CCS testing with an on-site laboratory, do you see Zouves Fertility participating in or pursuing any research?

Dr. Christo Zouves: We are constantly evaluating our results and using these results to implement new protocols and also to direct which embryos to transfer. It is difficult to do research incorporating randomized controlled trials within a private practice and it is also difficult to convince patients to be randomized possibly to a placebo treatment when the biological clock is ticking.

Karen Reynolds, LAc, MS, RN:
What are your thoughts about in vitro maturation?

Dr. Christo Zouves: I have been doing IVF for more than 30 years. What we found with the in vitro maturation process in the 90s was that there was so much more laboratory work required and not a lot of return as far as successful pregnancy. Some people like it as an option because there are fewer medications used and it could be seen as saving money. However, it is so much more work for the lab that no one can adequately fund it. It can be an option for women with PCOS {polycystic ovary syndrome} in which the resting follicle count can be in excess of 20. I still believe that the best results are obtained with some degree of stimulation and the retrieval of eggs that have been matured in the follicle rather that in the laboratory.

Karen Reynolds, LAc, MS, RN:
Thank you to you, Dr. Zouves, as well as to your staff for your time and kind sharing of your clinical expertise with me and for the benefit of my readers!

IN CLOSING

It has been a labor of love to create this book, and I hope you have found useful information here. For your reference I have added a Glossary of Genetic Terms after this section. Please see my blog at KReynoldsAcupuncture.com for weekly posts involving fertility, complimentary health topics as well as upcoming books to be released, such as my next one, which shall focus upon genetic topics for adult screening.

There is the saying "it takes a village," and it is not only applicable to the raising of children. It is also a necessity for authors so that they do not lose their minds. Many profound thanks to:

my husband Jim, for his never-ending support;

my copy editor Lynn Eder, who has kept this endeavor from being a giant mess, leder@ederedits.com/ ;

my multitalented and always tasteful graphic designer, Kelly Cazzaniga of Cazzaniga Design http://cazdesignstudio.com/;

my friend and local artist Rich Sigberman, who is a gifted painter and illustrator, not just a creator caricatures http://www.sigsart.com/;

Dr. Christo Zouves (http://www.goivf.com/) and genetics counselor Amy Vance (http://www.bayareagc.com/BAGC/home.html/) for their generous interview time, expertise and information;

and Kathy Colaiacovo, IT guru and voice of reason from her Nova Scotia based virtual assistant company Time on Task. http://timeontaskva.com/.

My wish for you the reader is a happy and healthy family,

the many blessings and benefits of the scientific age in which we live,

and of course what your heart holds dear.

Karen Reynolds, L.Ac., M.S., R.N.

Corte Madera, CA May 24, 2015.

GLOSSARY OF GENETIC TERMS

Aneuploidy

Here we have a bit of math and bit of genetics. It is easier to define aneuploidy by a comparison.

Eggs produced by women and sperm produced by men are described as *haploid*, which means they have exactly half of the number of chromosomes for a healthy human. An egg which is haploid contributes 23 genes, and a sperm which is haploid contributes 23 genes, so the resulting embryo will have a healthy total of 46 chromosomes. In contrast, for the purposes of reproductive medicine, aneuploid refers to an embryo, which has more or less than 46 total chromosomes. This is the case with children with Down syndrome, also known as trisomy 21. Because Down individuals have an extra chromosome at number 21, they carry a total of 47 chromosomes. This is why Down individuals have a characteristically shorter stature with broad facial features and oftentimes developmental delays or challenges in learning.

Array CGH (Also known as microarray-based comparative genomic hybridization)

Why is this testing more precise and more desirable from the perspective of fertility? The reality is that CGH offers more detailed and refined genetic information, which in turn will more accurately forecast if an embryo is genetically normal and likely to produce a healthy child. CGH can also be used for screening for suspected genetic disorders.

For those of you interested in the technical side of things, here is a bit on how it is conducted and why it works. As I've said, the DNA within our chromosomes—the road map for the body to develop—is shaped like a two strands of ribbon precisely twisting together. This is often referred to as a double helix shape or the spiraling ladder shape. The twisting happens because there is a stickiness or affinity for parts along the length of the ribbons. Remember that DNA is made of four different components (or bases): adenine (A), thymine (T), guanine (G), and cytosine (C). Adenine will always stick with or pair with only thymine. Guanine will always stick with or pair with only cytosine.

It is somewhat like magnets sticking together. With magnets, the North and South Poles bond together easily and tightly, but if you try put two North Poles together or two South Poles together, there is resistance and they do not "fit." The twists and turns of DNA strands happen because the adenine on one ribbon searches out and sticks to the Thymine on the other ribbon. The same affinity happens for the guanine and cytosine along the ribbons. Adenine will always be like a magnet for thymine, and guanine will always be like a magnet for cytosine.

So why am I describing this? One how-it-works aspect of the microarray-based comparative genomic hybridization (CGH) involves a slide or "chip." The chip is prepared with strands of normal (also known as "reference") DNA dyed a specific color and placed next to strands of the patient's DNA, which is dyed a different specific color. Similar to the North and

South Poles of magnets which pull together when close to one another, the strands of the reference DNA will "hybridise" or stick together with the strands of the patient's DNA.

Once the hybridization or coiling of the strands is complete, the chip is placed in a microarry scanner machine. This step is somewhat like art class as in mixing of primary colors to make various shades. Red plus green makes yellow. If the testing or reference DNA is green and the patient's DNA is red we would expect a specific color of yellow to be produced. The scanner very precisely measures the color distribution. Too much red would mean there is extra genetic material from the patient, which might mean extra chromosomes or a genetic duplication, such as those that occur with Down syndrome. Too much green would mean that the patient's DNA is missing genetic material.

Autosomal Dominant Disorder

- A person has inherited only one copy of a gene associated with a genetic disorder
- Usually one parent has the genetic disease associated with the gene in question
- 50% of children born will carry a autosomal dominant gene *but* there are often lower rates of actual disease development

Examples are familial hypercholesterolemia, Huntington's disease, Marfan syndrome, and colorectal cancer.

Autosomal Recessive Disorder

- A person has inherited two copies of a gene associated with a genetic disorder

- Frequently (but not always) both parents do not have signs or symptoms of a disease but simply are "carriers" for the genetic disease. Many autosomal recessive diseases can skip multiple generations, meaning no family suffers from a disease or show signs of illness. However, they still carry the gene for it and it can be passed to children. This illustrates another reason why genetic testing is so very important.
- 25% of children born will carry the autosomal recessive disorder

Examples are cystic fibrosis, Tay-Sachs disease, sickle cell disorder, spinal muscular atrophy, Niemann-Pick disease

Chromosomes

Chromosomes are thread-like structures floating in the nucleus (the more central, dense area) of your cells. They hold genes lined up in a specific order. Chromosomes are the delicate strands of specialized tissue in your cells, which carry your specific DNA—your genetic blueprints. The chromosomes hold the road maps, which guide our bodies through the trip of normal growth and development. They dictate everything from obvious characteristics like our eye color or height but more importantly we now know they determine what diseases or physical tendencies may unfold for us in life. Within the context of reproductive medicine, examination of chromosomes gives us highly valuable information about an embryo being likely to transform into a healthy child and/or future health or probability of inherited disorders.

The normal number of chromosomes within our cells is 46. These are arranged in pairs and numbered from 1 to 22. With respect to the 1 to 22, we inherit a gene from each parent to make 44. The remaining 2 genes are called sex chromosomes.

Females have an XX set of sex chromosomes (one X contributed from the mother and one X contributed from the father). Males have XY set of sex chromosomes (one X contributed from the mother and one Y contributed from the father). Women's eggs can only pass on an X chromosome to their children, whereas a man's sperm can pass on either an X chromosome or a Y chromosome depending upon the sperm itself, which fertilizes the egg.

DNA

DNA is abbreviation for the giant scientific term deoxyribonucleic acid. DNA is the hereditary material of all living things. There is DNA in plants, in animals, in microscopic organisms and essentially all living things, but of course the instructions are different in each type of living being. You may have heard DNA described as a ladder-like structure, except the ladder twists as opposed to staying straight. The "rungs" of the ladder are compromised always of 2 of 4 possible base pairs. These bases are called adenine (A), thymine (T), guanine (G), and cytosine (C). Adenine will always stick with or pair with only Thymine. Guanine will always stick with or pair with only cytosine. In his book, *The Language of Life,* Dr. Francis Collins (page 6) estimates there are 3.1 billion "rungs" on the human DNA ladder. So there is a mind-boggling amount of genetic information existing in each of our bodies.

Gene

A gene is a segment or section of a DNA ladder that carries a specific collection of instructions. Genes can hold problematic (also known as mutated) instructions for example: the ones which code the proteins for the cystic fibrosis transmembrane conductance regulator gene (CTFR). Changes in this gene's protein are known to produce cystic fibrosis, which is a genetically inherited disease. The good thing is that we can test for the present of mutations within your CTFR gene and many others. Should you happen to be a carrier for the gene mutation, there are measures that can be taken to test to see if it is passed to an embryo or fetus. If you are seeking to become pregnant or undergoing assisted reproductive assistance to do so, this is one small illustration of the giant value of genetic testing.

Genome

The entirety of your genetic material is your genome. Here is where terms may begin to get fuzzy. Think of your genome as your own very large, private book. Your chromosomes are tidy, vertical chapters inside your book. Your genes are the pages within each chapter and your DNA are your words upon each page. Essentially each baby inherits half of its "book" from the mother and half of its "book" from the father.

Karyotyping

Karyotyping is an older version of genetic testing in which chromosomes are stained and viewed under a high power microscope. Up close, chromosomes have a short end and long end. They are joined between the long and short ends by what is called a centromere, somewhat like an organic waistband. Historically, scientists examined the series of stripes along chromosomes as they marched out from the centromere to the ends of the chromosomes. It was evident when stripes did not identically match in pairs or if there were added or missing stripes. The problem with this method is that sometimes the changes in the stripes are too small to be seen even with a high quality laboratory microscope and an experienced clinician. This problem spurred development of what is called the microarray-based comparative genomic hybridization (CGH) form of testing, also known as Array CGH.

Mitochondrial aka maternal inheritance

- Involves genetic material in maternal mitochondria DNA
- Maternal eggs contribute mitochondria to a growing embryo
- Only women can pass this to their offspring

Examples include Leber's hereditary optic neuropathy

Mosaicism

Mosaicism is the situation in which cells within your system may not all be genetically identical. These are abnormalities quite common to egg and sperm cell in your body, and it is also quite common to see mosaicsim appear during the cellular divisions in the early days of development following egg fertilization with sperm.

Single gene disorders

These are disorders in which one gene has mutated. There are quite a few variables with respect to types of single gene disorders, how they may be inherited, and how they may affect offspring. Please see below.

X-linked dominant

- A person has inherited a mutation specifically on the X-chromosome

- Overall these are more rare diseases, but can be devastating when they do occur
- For men with male offspring: male children will be unaffected because males will inherit only the Y chromosome from the father
- For men with female offspring, all female children will have the disorder
- For women: 50% of all offspring will inherit the disorder

Examples are X-linked hypophosphatemic rickets, incontinentia pigmenti type 2, Aicardi syndrome, and rare cases of males with Klinefelter syndrome

X-linked recessive

- Individuals with X-linked genetic disorders have mutations on the X-chromosome
- Men are more generally more affected by X-linked recessive genetic disorders than women
- For a man with male offspring: male children will be unaffected because males will inherit only the Y chromosome from the father
- For a man with female offspring: all female children will carry one copy of the mutated gene
- For a woman, 50% of chance of having sons affected by the genetic mutation and 50% of having daughters who are carriers of the genetic mutation

Examples are hemophila A, Duchenne muscular dystrophy, red-green color blindness, muscular atrophy, androgenetic alopecia

Y-linked

- Individuals with Y-linked genetic disorders have mutations on the Y chromosome
- All male offspring will be affected because males inherit only the Y chromosome from the father
- No female offspring will be affected because females inherit only an X chromosome from their fathers

Examples are male infertility, hypertrichosis pinnae

Endnotes

1 Kohane IS, Masys DR, Altman RB. The incidentalome: A threat to genomic medicine [published erratum appears in JAMA 2006;296:1466]. JAMA 2006;296:212–5.

2 Collins, FS. *The Language of Life: DNA and the Revolution in Personalized Medicine. New York: HarperCollins Publishers, 2010, 44*

3 http://www.helpthals.org/blog/wp-content/uploads/2015/03/TSF-Dr.-Coates-April-18th-2015.pdf

4 http://ghr.nlm.nih.gov/condition/sickle-cell-disease

5 Collins, 49

6 My testing options, Spinal Muscular Atrophy Carrier Testing:
https://www.labcorp.com/wps/portal/!ut/p/c1/04_SB8K8xLLM9
MSSzPy8xBz9CP0os3h_U2cv30B_IwP3ADMnA09Dc38L50B
TQ_dgQ6B8JJK8f4C5gYFnaJiJS0hggJFZiDkB3X4e-bmp-gW5
EeUAKliSng!!/dl2/d1/L0lDU0lKSWdrbUEhIS9JRFJBQUlpQ
2dBek15cXchL1lCSkoxTkExTkk1MC01RncvN19PNUNKTV
FPMjBHTzcwMEkxRkQwSjRWMUtJNS9JX19fXzE!/?WCM_
PORTLET=PC_7_O5CJMQO20GO700I1FD0J4V1KI5_
WCM&WCM_GLOBAL_CONTEXT=/wps/wcm/connect/
mtoLib/reproductive/home/testing/tests+by+name/spinal+
muscular+atrophy+carrier+testing (May 20, 2015).

7 http://www.reuters.com/article/2010/03/15/us-screening-fatal-disease-costly-idUSTRE62E2A820100315

8 Collins, 48

9 Musci TJ. Fragile X Syndrome: Carrier Screening in the Prenatal Population, [https://www.genome.gov/Pages/About/OD/ReportsPublications/Feb2008_CarrierScreening_Musci.pdf]

10 http://www.mayomedicallaboratories.com/test-catalog/Clinical+and+Interpretive/87857

11 http://www.mayoclinic.org/diseases-conditions/down-syndrome/basics/causes/con-20020948

12 http://www.marchofdimes.com/professionals/14332_15455.asp

13 Committee Opinion, College Practice Bulletin 88, Number 545, Invasive Prenatal Testing for Aneuploidy, The American College of Obstetricians and Gynecologists Committee on Genetics The Society for Maternal-Fetal Medicine, http://www.acog.org/Resources-And-Publications/Committee-Opinions/Committee-on-Genetics/Noninvasive-Prenatal-Testing-for-Fetal-Aneuploidy, December 2012.

14 National Organization for Rare Disorders, Rare Disease Information, http://rarediseases.org/for-patients-and-families/information-resources/rare-disease-information/(May 20, 2015).

15 Committee Opinion, Number 581, The Use of Chromosomal Microarray Analysis in Prenatal Diagnosis, The American College of Obstetricians and Gynecologists Committee on Genetics The Society for Maternal-Fetal Medicine, http://www.acog.org/Resources-And-Publications/Committee-Opinions/Committee-on-Genetics/The-Use-of-Chromosomal-Microarray-Analysis-in-Prenatal-Diagnosis, December 2013.

16 ACOG Committee Opinion Number 410, Ethical Issues in Genetic Testing, Committee on Ethics, Committee on Genetics, http://www.acog.org/Resources_And_Publications/Committee_Opinions/Committee_on_Ethics/Ethical_Issues_in_Genetic_Testing, June 2008.

17 Ibid.

18 http://www.forbes.com/sites/roberthof/2014/06/20/seven-months-after-fda-slapdown-23andme-returns-with-new-health-report-submission/

19 Shangwu C, Fengjuan LV, Jie G, Jianghai L, Zehuan L, Younggui F, Anlong X. HLA Class II polymorphisms associated with the physiologic characteristics defined by traditional Chinese medicine: Linking modern genetics with an ancient medicine. *Journal of Alternative and Complementary Medicine*. 2007 13 (2), 231-239.

20 Chang SY, Hi JP, Joo-Ho C, Hye-Jung L, Byung-Cheol L. Genome-wide association study of the four-constitution medicine. *Journal of Alternative and Complementary Medicine*. 2009; 15(12), 1327-133.

21 Morgan, K. K., (2014). Patterns of Disease. *Genome*, Summer Fall 2014, 38-47.

22 Capalbo A, Rienzi L, Cimadomo D, Maggiulli R, Elliott T, Wright G, Zsolt PN and Upaldi FM. Correlation between standard blastocyst morphology, euploidy and implantation: an observational study in two centers involving 956 screened blastocysts. *The Journal of Human Reproduction* (2014) 29 (6): 1173-1181:1178.

23 Scott Jr. RT, Upham KM, Forman EJ, Hong KH, Scott KL, Taylor D, Tao X, and Treff NR. Blastocyst biopsy with comprehensive chromosome screening and fresh embryo transfer significantly increases in vitro fetilization implantation and delivery rates: a randomized controlled trial. *Fertility and Sterility* Vol. 100, No. 3, September 2013 0015-0282:998.

Printed in Dunstable, United Kingdom

91222517R00067